Pescatarian Cookbook for Beginners

Mouth-Watering, Easy and Healthy Pescatarian Recipes to Delight the Senses and Nourish Your Body

By Deborah Patterson

Legal & Disclaimer

The information contained in this book and its contents is not designed to replace or take the place of any form of medical or professional advice; and is not meant to replace the need for independent medical, financial, legal or other professional advice or services, as may be required. The content and information in this book has been provided for educational and entertainment purposes only.

The content and information contained in this book has been compiled from sources deemed reliable, and it is accurate to the best of the Author's knowledge, information and belief. However, the Author cannot guarantee its accuracy and validity and cannot be held liable for any errors and/or omissions. Further, changes are periodically made to this book as and when needed. Where appropriate and/or necessary, you must consult a professional (including but not limited to your doctor, attorney, financial advisor or such other professional advisor) before using any of the suggested remedies, techniques, or information in this book.

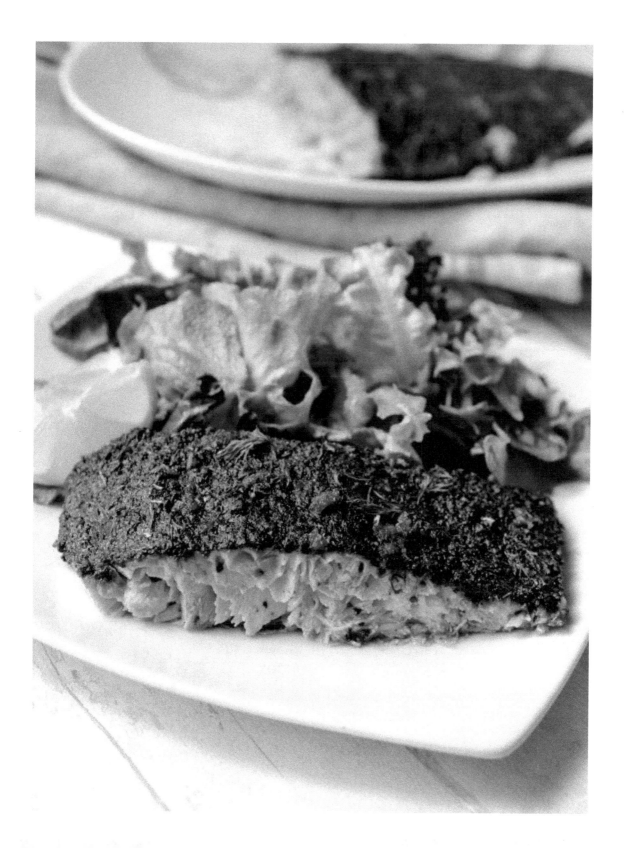

CONTENT

Introduction

Pescatarian eating is often considered a branch of vegetarianism, and, depending on personal preference, one may include eggs and dairy products in their regimen. The Pescatarian Plan incorporates lots of vegetables, fruits, whole grains, healthy fats, not too much sugar, and seafood, without red meat and poultry. The fish provides the omega-3 fats our bodies need meanwhile; red meat promotes the diseases that fish helps protect from us. And poultry has its issues such as salmonella and the unfair treatment of chickens. Introducing fish and seafood into your meals can be one of many ways to improve the overall quality of your diet, all while embracing conscious eating and nutrition. It's important to realize that the food you eat can deliver these compelling benefits, allowing you to live up to your maximum potential.

The recipes in this book are plant-forward, fiber-rich, fish, and seafood dishes with a balance of foods from the land and sea. In this cookbook, I will show you many ways to get creative in the kitchen. I also wanted to showcase how to transform familiar ingredients into unique and exciting dishes inspired by global cuisines. In addition to the 80 delectable and healthy recipes, you will learn about this diet, how to turn your kitchen into a pescatarian haven, and how to find and maintain your healthy weight naturally.

Not a pescatarian? Don't worry; you don't have to be one to reap the benefits of this cookbook. This book will help you make a smooth transition to pescatarian cooking and eating, putting your best health quickly within your grasp. Anyone can benefit from adopting this diet, whether you are already on this diet, aspiring to be on this diet, a vegetarian who wants to start including fish, or someone who eats everything.

Lastly, remember that everything compiled in this book has been through research and the experiences of individuals, so feel free to question what you read in this book. It is encouraged that you do your research on the things you want to look in-depth. If nothing else, I hope these recipes inspire you to try something different or find a new way to connect with your food.

Let's get cooking!

Chapter-1 Pescatarian Diet Primer

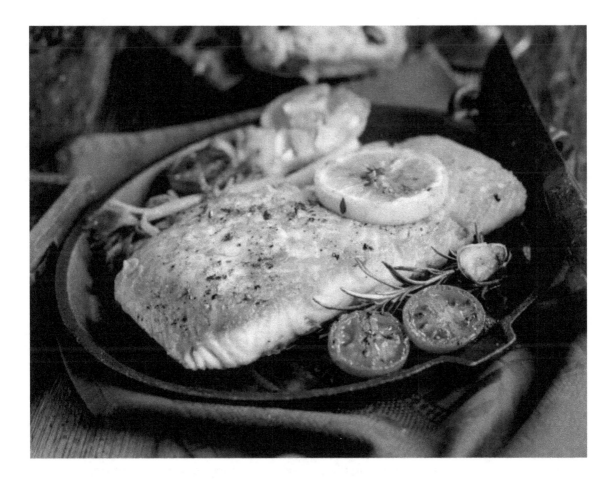

What is Pescatarian Diet

The term pescatarian derives from the combination of the words "pesce" and "vegetarian" (a person who eats a diet consisting of vegetables). "Pesce" comes from the Italian language, meaning fish.

The pescatarian diet contains fruits, vegetables, whole grains, nuts, legumes, produce, healthy fats, seafood, and sometimes dairy and eggs. A pescatarian diet lowers the risk of having chronic medical problems, such as heart disease. Seafood generally has a lower amount of fat and cholesterol than most meats, which is beneficial to the health of your heart.

So many reasons would push a person to go on a pescatarian diet. It could be because of an ethical or moral stance, wherein a person's culture prohibits the eating of warm-blooded creatures. Environmental concerns and treatment of animals are some of the reasons people pursue a pescatarian diet. Some people also disagree with poor labor conditions and go on this diet for humanitarian reasons. The reasons include:

- Not wanting to partake in killing animals for food

- Disagreeing with inhumane factory practices

- Not wanting to support the poor labor conditions that workers experience

- Disagreeing with the land and resource use for animal feed and production because it is unjust.

The pescatarian diet can also be an excellent way to transition if you are aiming to become a vegetarian someday. It is because you will still eat seafood until you can eliminate all animal meat from your diet. Turning to a pescatarian diet is challenging to do overnight, and the process of slow change will not be easy. However, if you want to take this route, whatever your reason, then you can get there with an understanding of your nutritional needs and a solid game plan.

It's more flexible than a vegetarian or vegan diet: The vegan diet calls for the exclusion of all animal products—even honey. There are multiple versions of the vegetarian diet; some versions include dairy and eggs, and others don't. What all variations of the vegetarian diet have in common is the exclusion of animal flesh. When following a pescatarian diet, you will have greater flexibility than when following a vegan or vegetarian diet. You'll have the freedom to choose from healthy protein sources, like fish, seafood, eggs, and dairy. It makes it easier to get dense but lean protein, vitamins, minerals, and healthy fats.

The Pescatarian Diet and Your Health

Although few studies isolate a pescatarian diet to examine health benefits, and many of these studies on individual nutrients are available. Omega-3 fatty acids are among the most exceptionally studied nutrients of all, so we have a decent comprehension of the role they play in human well-being.

Here's how some of the science breaks down when it comes to these topics:

Omega-3s

These fatty acids are a type of unsaturated fat. Although also found in nuts and seeds, the omega 3 found in animals and especially seafood is the best for human consumption. Omega-3s from low-mercury seafood can also support a healthy pregnancy and brain and neurodevelopment in infants and children.

Mercury

You can find mercury in low or trace amounts in most fish. It accumulates in the flesh of the fish when they ingest it from their diet. When ingested in high amounts, it can also accumulate in humans and lead to neurotoxic effects. However, the guidelines to consume eight to 12 ounces of fish per week are as safe levels of intake.

Dairy

The inclusion of dairy in a pescatarian or plant-based diet is optional. For those with lactose intolerance or dairy allergies, it is best to eliminate dairy or find low-lactose or dairy-free alternatives to replace traditional dairy products. Dairy can play a decisive role in human health, providing essential nutrients such as calcium, potassium, phosphorus, vitamins A, D, and B12, riboflavin, and niacin. Research shows that including low-fat dairy in your diet may prevent osteoporosis and fractures, reduce the risk of type 2 diabetes, and potentially lower the risk of heart diseases.

Fish

Omega-3 fats—which have anti-inflammatory benefits—are essential to our health and abundant in only a few foods, fish being one of them. To ensure you are consuming sufficient omega-3s is to eat a variety of fish, especially fatty fish. Omega-3s Come from the Sea. These super healthy fats can vary according to the type of fish and whether the fish was farm-raised or wild-caught. Wild-caught fish acquire and accumulate omega-3s in their tissue when they eat phytoplankton that consume microalgae. Farmed fish receive them if they are f fortified with omega-3s. The pescatarian diet, along with exercise, sleep, and stress reduction, works together to crush chronic inflammation.

Fattier fish, like salmon, mackerel, sardines, tuna, and herring, contain higher amounts of omega-3s than leaner fish, like tilapia, bass, and cod. Eating fish protects your heart. Eating fish lowers your risk of heart disease, lowers your triglycerides, and lowers your blood pressure. The research on the benefits of omega-3 found that men who ate fish twice a week after surviving a heart attack had a 29 percent reduction compared with men who did not eat fish. It's not surprising that populations that consume a lot of fish, like in Japan and certain Mediterranean regions, have fewer heart attacks.

One of the most common questions regarding fish consumption is "What about mercury?" This concern stems from the fact that several recent industrial activities release mercury into the air. A portion of these pollutants settles in the world's waterways and results in trace levels of mercury in the fish we eat. These levels, though, are not enough to warrant avoiding fish.

Below are three recommendations to maximize the benefits of eating fish while minimizing risk:

1. Avoid shark, swordfish, king mackerel, bigeye tuna, and tilefish.

2. Eat common fish varieties that are low in mercury, such as salmon, canned light tuna, trout, and catfish.

Plant-based Protein and Benefits

Chronic diseases, for example, cancer, and heart disease, is unfortunately all too common in the United States. There's good evidence that changing our diet can help prevent chronic diseases. A diet rich in red meat and poultry has a direct link to some significant health complications, including heart disease and diabetes. It has sparked a growing public interest in a plant-based diet that helps protect us from these same chronic diseases.

The pescatarian diet encompasses plant foods, like fruits, veggies, whole grains, and legumes. All these are rich in antioxidants and polyphenols—potent, health-boosting plant compounds.

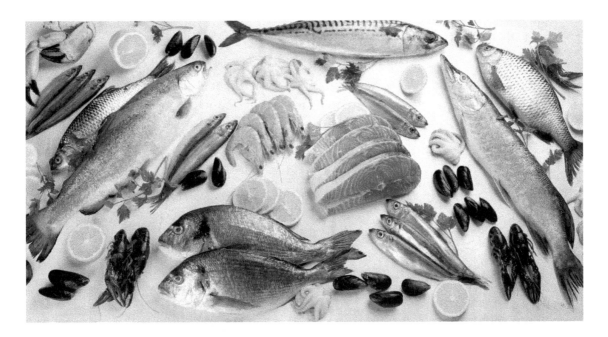

There are lots of other potential health benefits of eating more plant-based food.

Below are some of the benefits:

- **Energy boost**

Plant-based foods are full of nutrients that fuel energy levels, and many people find they have more sustained energy levels throughout the day.

- **Immune boost**

The nutrients your immune system needs to be strong are plentiful in plants. Focus on the dark green, red, and orange fruits and vegetables, plus seeds for zinc. Better digestion. With a massive boost in fiber, most people find their digestion improves.

- **Soothed stomach**

Overeating meat, dairy, processed foods, and fatty foods can all cause your stomach to act up and lead to heartburn and indigestion.

- **Faster recovery after workouts**

Athletes, runners, and bodybuilders on plant-based diets report that they recover faster after workouts, meaning they can fit in more training than their omnivorous counterparts. It may be due to increased antioxidants, vitamins, potassium, or a decrease in the inflammatory compounds found in meat and dairy.

10 Plant Super-foods

It's easy to get enough protein from plant-based foods, and it's equally important to know what foods pack the most significant protein punch.

Here are some of the top protein foods compatible with the pescatarian diet. Some of these foods in the table aren't meat substitutes; they are just healthy protein sources to add to many dishes.

Chia Seeds		These seeds are rich in fatty acids (omega-3) and calcium, which help maintain healthy bones, minimize muscle cramps, and aid sleep.
Quinoa, Amaranth, and Teff		High in protein, an excellent alternative to beans if they give you gas. They have high levels of quercetin and kaempferol than other foods—both compounds help limit the inflammatory response to allergens.
Avocados		The fat from avocados is mostly monounsaturated, which are shown to lower the risk of heart disease and reduce blood levels of LDL cholesterol.

Chickpeas		They have a complex carbohydrate for energy, as well as a protein source, which helps muscles, digestion, hormones, and detoxification. Not only are chickpeas a super versatile ingredient, but they also contain 6 grams of protein per ½-cup serving. They also have a specific type of fiber that results in better blood fat regulation, lower levels of LDL cholesterol, and insulin secretion.
Nuts and seeds		Like sunflower seeds, almonds, or walnuts are a heart-healthy snack. You can also use them as toppings on oatmeal and salads, and even in sandwiches.
Tempeh		Tempeh is made up of fermented soybeans, and it's less processed than tofu. A 3-ounce serving contains 16 grams of protein and just 140 calories.

Lentils		Lentils contain 9 grams of protein per ½-cup serving.
Edamame		Whether you enjoy them in a stir-fry or a salad, these baby soybeans have 9 grams of protein per ½ cup.
Black beans		Supplies nearly 8 grams of protein per ½-cup serving
Hemp seeds		I often sprinkle these on my yogurt bowls or smoothies, because three tablespoons of hemp seeds contain 10 grams of protein.

The Principles of Pescatarian Diet

If you're new to a pescatarian lifestyle, there are several vital components to remember, which are listed below.

1. Fish and Seafood as Primary Animal Proteins:

A pescatarian diet includes fresh and saltwater fish, shellfish, and crustaceans. You won't find meat such as beef, pork, poultry, wild game, or other meats in this book.

2. The Ability to Include Eggs and Dairy:

Many Pescatarians choose to include eggs and dairy as protein sources. However, some prefer to rely solely on fish and seafood for animal protein. The best part about the pescatarian diet is that the choice is up to you.

3. Plant-Forward Focus:

The plant-forwardness of this diet encourages you to consume a variety of filling and nutrient-rich fruits, veggies, whole grains, nuts, seeds, beans, and other legumes. This diet is mostly plant-based, meaning plant-based foods should take up most of your plate. At least half of your plate should be made up of vegetables at most meals. It comes out to about two handfuls of greens or about 2 cups at each meal.

4. Lots of Fruits and Vegetables:

A pescatarian diet encourages a high intake of fruits and vegetables. These are nutrient-rich ingredients that provide many essential vitamins and minerals, as well as beneficial antioxidants and phytochemicals for health.

5. Whole Grains and Fiber-Rich Foods:

A pescatarian diet is not meant to be a low-carbohydrate diet. It includes carbohydrates from whole grains and other starchy or fiber-rich foods such as potatoes, legumes, and ancient grains. Fiber-Rich: The fiber richness of this lifestyle will keep you full and satisfied. Your focus should be on whole grains, complex carbohydrates, and of course, tons of fruits and vegetables to reap the benefits of fiber.

6. Healthy Fats and lean proteins:

Olive oil, avocados, nuts, and seeds are included in this diet because they contain healthy fats. These plant-based fats are mostly composed of monounsaturated fats, a type of fat that has been shown to have heart-protective properties. Most fish and other seafood are naturally lean, making it easy to choose heart-healthy proteins. Fattier kinds of fish contain healthy fats that you can find in a minimal selection of foods. The fats in fish make this one of the most heart-healthy diets out there.

7. Properly Portioned and Balanced:

Understanding the portion sizes and safe seafood intake in a pescatarian diet is essential. A well-rounded pescatarian diet will have the correct portions of protein (25%), grains/carbs (25%), and fruits and vegetables (50%).

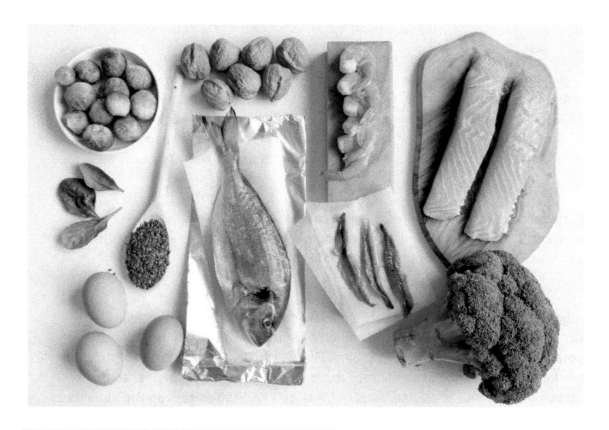

Benefits of A Pescatarian Diet

- **Fiber:**

Our bodies work better when we eat enough fiber. Sufficient fiber intake of 25 to 38 grams has been shown to improve digestion, lower cholesterol and blood pressure, reduce food cravings, and boost satiety. With so many fruits, vegetables, whole grains, and legumes, a pescatarian diet is usually higher in fiber than a typical American diet. It can support good gut health, which often helps with improved regularity or a decrease in uncomfortable GI-related symptoms.

- **It's lower in saturated fat:**

A pescatarian diet is usually lower in saturated fat. Fish has only tiny amounts of saturated fats, also known as bad fats. Animal protein, on the other hand—particularly in red meat and the dark meat of poultry—contributes to higher amounts of saturated fats. Replacing saturated fats with the healthy fats found in fish has been linked to a decreased risk of heart disease.

- **It's great for weight loss:**

When done the right way and in the right portions, foods that make up this diet can help you lose weight—and keep it off!

- **It helps lower your carbon footprint:**

 The consumption of meat—especially red meat—is a significant contributor to harmful greenhouse gases. Avoiding meat, eating more plant-based foods, and including the right amount of fish are a win-win for both your health and the environment.

- **You'll feel happier:**

Living the pescatarian lifestyle will put a pep in your step. The proper amount of nutrients, along with the balance of exercise, sleep, and stress management will do wonders for your mood, energy level, and overall happiness.

- **It's a brilliant choice for your brain:**

No other organ in the human body is fatter than the brain. The essential omega-3 fatty acids found in fish are considered critical for healthy brain development in children and maintaining optimal brain health later in life. Even during pregnancy, it's known that omega-3s offer enormous benefits to your baby's brain development. Brain Health The brain is affected by the types of dietary fat a person consumes than any other body organ, except perhaps the heart.

- **Lower Blood Pressure:**

Eating fish and seafood frequently has been related to lower blood pressure in adults, which reduces the risk of heart disease. Research shows fish in this diet has been shown to decrease triglyceride levels.

- **Satiety and Satisfaction:**

The combination of protein, fat, and fiber helps you feel full after eating, which may help alleviate hunger between meals and reduce fluctuations in energy levels. When following a pescatarian diet, these nutrients are present in most meals in balanced ratios, helping you walk away from meals feeling truly satisfied.

- **Sustainability and Practicality:**

A pescatarian diet is very flexible and can be easily adapted based on your tastes and preferences. Evidence shows that restrictive diets are not sustainable in the long term. Having more choices means you might be more successful at creating a realistic lifestyle you can maintain without feeling deprived.

- **Complete Nutrition:**

Vegan and vegetarian diets that eliminate all or most animal products can create nutrition gaps, leading to potential health concerns. A pescatarian diet that includes fish and seafood, as well as the option for eggs and dairy, is a more flexible approach that offers good or excellent sources of essential nutrients.

- **It fights aging in every single way.**

By fending off chronic inflammation, helping keep arteries clear, and dousing you with antioxidants, this diet protects your heart and helps stave off cancer, type 2 diabetes, and even erectile dysfunction.

FAQs about Pescatarian Diet

- **Can I lose weight on this plan?**

Weight is not a controllable behavior. We can, however, support good health by eating balanced, nourishing meals. Adopting a pescatarian diet as part of your lifestyle may lead to improvements in health and weight loss, but weight loss is not guaranteed or our primary goal. But I can tell you that this pescatarian way of eating is more comfortable to sustain over the long run than a low-fat or low-carb diet.

- **Can I have chicken, beef, pork, lamb, or other animal meats on this diet?**

Sure. But try not to. I'm leaving the meat out because my goal is to present the hands-down healthiest way of eating. If you want to eat these foods on occasion, go ahead.

- **Why is red meat not recommended?**

Red meat of any type relates to higher rates of heart disease, cancer, and premature death. As for poultry, there are both nutritional and ethical issues. If you eat the poultry skin, you get a mouthful of artery-clogging saturated fat. And low-fat turkey and chicken deli meats are loaded with sodium and cancer-causing nitrites.

- **Is sugar allowed on this plan?**

It is—but in moderation, as eaten in long-lived cultures like those along the Mediterranean Sea.

- **Do I have to eat seafood every day?**

No. The current recommendation for adults is two to three servings per week (totaling eight to 12 ounces). A pescatarian diet does not require you to include seafood at every meal; in fact, the majority of your meals could be plant-based.

- **Isn't seafood expensive?**

These recipes include affordable options that are easy to find in most grocery stores. Some types of seafood can be quite expensive, but these recipes concentrate on fresh or frozen fillets of commonly available fish or canned options for tuna and salmon. And if you start preparing more meals at home—you'll save a bundle over eating out.

- **I don't live anywhere near water. Can I still do this diet?**

Definitely—you need a discerning eye (and nose) to ensure that the "fresh" seafood is just that.

- **Is a pescatarian diet safe?**

A pescatarian diet is safe for most people, so long as you're aware of which fish contain high levels of mercury. Generally, the higher the fish appears on the food chain, the higher the mercury content. Some of the highest-mercury fish include swordfish, shark, king mackerel, and tilefish. Pregnant women should also avoid raw fish to reduce the risk of foodborne illness.

- **Do I have to include eggs or dairy?**

Many people who identify as pescatarians include eggs and dairy, but it is a personal choice. There are limitations for someone with lactose intolerance or an allergy to eggs or dairy. In those cases, you can use many alternative products in recipes as a replacement, such as nuts or coconut milk.

- **Does cooking take lots of time?**

You can make any of the recipes in 30 minutes or less. If you have even less time, look for the Quick Prep label for meals that require little or no active cooking and take 10 minutes or less to prepare.

- **How do I know the pescatarian diet is the right diet for me?**

It is the perfect plan for you if you are trying to avoid red meat and poultry or want to include more fish and plants in your diet. You should develop more of a pescatarian diet if you want a food that is energizing, satisfying, anti-inflammatory, and heart protective.

Chapter-2 Pescatarian Action Plan

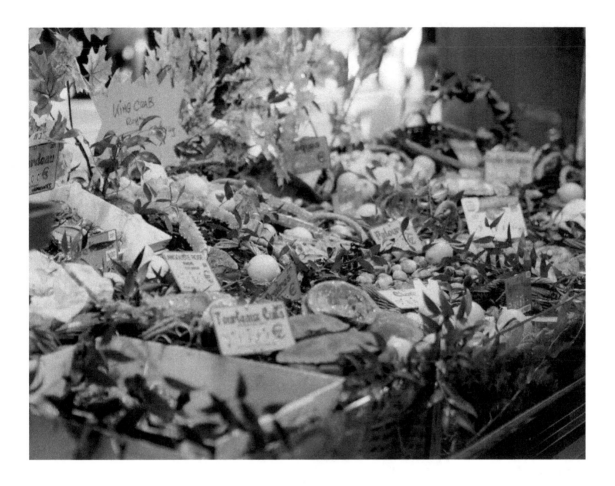

Shopping

Making the perfect seafood recipe starts with selecting the perfect seafood. The following is a compilation of tips from the U.S. Food and Drug Administration, Environmental Defense Fund, and good old common sense. The process starts by buying seafood from a retailer who follows proper food handling practices. It helps ensure that the seafood you are purchasing is safe and high quality.

Picking Fresh Seafood

The key to buying perfect seafood is only to buy fish that is refrigerated or properly iced.

- **Assess your kitchen and take inventory.**

Before purchasing a single ingredient, I like to scan my fridge, pantry, and freezer to account for what I already have. This way, you can avoid purchasing too much, and you'll make sure you have room to store everything once you get it back home.

- **Plan your schedule.**

If you know you'll be cooking your fish or seafood in the next day or so, purchasing fresh is a great option. However, if you need to wait longer, it might be preferable to buy frozen seafood so you can thaw it when you're ready to cook.

- **Inspection**

Inspect the fillet to ensure there are no separations or cracks in the flesh. When gently poked, the flesh should be firm, and the indentation from your finger should spring back to its original shape. Flesh that is mushy or soft and remains dented from your finger is a sign that the fish is old. For whole fish, the skin should be firm, shiny, metallic, and moist. Check the gills to ensure they are pinkish red. The eyes should be moist, clear, and slightly bulging. Avoid eyes that are discolored, cloudy, or sunken.

- **Smell the fish.**

If it smells fishy, it's not fresh. Fresh fish should never have a strong fishy smell. You should expect a salty, briny smell since it's from the ocean.

- **Check the color of the fillet**

Fish fillets should have no patches, discoloration, or drying around the edges. If visible, the veins of the fish should appear red, not gray or dark brown. Only red-fleshed fish, such as tuna, will have dark veins.

- **Mussels and Clams**

When buying mussels and clams, look to make sure shells are not cracked or discolored. Most of the shells should close. If any of them are open, a slight tap on the shell should close it, ensuring that the creature is alive. Discard shells that don't close when tapped. Always wash thoroughly. For mussels, scrub the outside of the shells and remove the beard. For clams, soak for 10 minutes in cold water, which will remove the salt inside. After being cooked, the clams and mussels should open. Discard ones that do not open.

- **For fresh fillets or steaks:**

Ask to touch the fish before purchasing or have the fishmonger do this for you. There should be some spring in the flesh, and it should appear moist and clean and show no discoloration or drying around the edges. If purchasing packaged fresh fish, examine the packaging to look for time and temperature indicators. It lets you know the fish was correctly handled and stored at the correct temperature.

- **For shellfish:**

Sacks or containers of fresh seafood should have a tag with a label. It will tell you how the shellfish were harvested and from where, and you can locate the processor's certification number to verify the safety and quality of the seafood if needed. Avoid or discard any oysters, clams, or mussels with cracked or broken shells.

- **When purchasing frozen:**

Use the same general rules for judging frozen fish based on appearance. Reach for packages that are toward the bottom or back of a freezer case because they are less likely to have experienced thawing and refreezing. Ice crystals inside the package aren't a good sign.

- **Canned, pouched, or preserved fish in tins:**

Read labels for information on how the seafood is packed (in water versus in oil) and the sustainability standards used for fishing. As with other food labels, it can be hard to distinguish the validity of labels that use vague terms like "wild-caught" or "sustainably caught." You're better off verifying the species and fishing methods to determine whether it is an ethical and environmentally friendly choice.

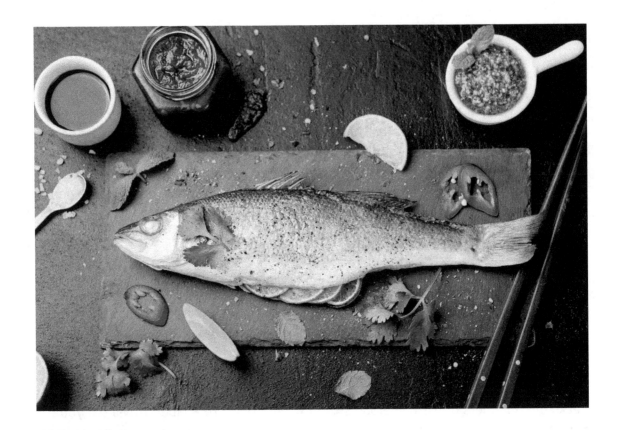

Cooking

Below are some conventional cooking methods that can get you great results with home cooking:

- **Pan Roasting:**

Pan roasting is similar to panfrying in that a shallow pan coated with oil serves as the cooking surface. It's considered a dry-heat method and can be a good option for fish or seafood, especially if preparing one-skillet meals or pan roasting other ingredients. Start with medium heat for evenly cooked fish that doesn't become too dry or flaky.

- **Oven Roasting:**

Roasting in the oven occurs at temperatures above 150ºF. It is also a dry-heat cooking method, meaning the flavor of the fish or seafood is enhanced while cooking without relying on a sauce, stew, or gravy. Start with oven temperatures around 350ºF, and make adjustments to time and temperature based on your recipe and the size of the fish you're preparing.

- **Poaching:**

Poaching uses a liquid to simmer the fish in a shallow pan. It can be a speedy cooking process, sometimes taking no more than 10 minutes. Poaching adds flavor without adding extra fat. It's a good fit for less oily whitefish, such as tilapia, cod, halibut, or snapper, but it could also work for salmon and trout. Use a slotted spatula or fish turner, as the cooked fish may easily flake apart in the poaching liquid.

- **Searing:**

Searing occurs over high heat on a flat surface. It creates a caramelized crust and, when done correctly, should not cause sticking or burning to the pan. Salmon, shrimp, tuna, and swordfish steaks are commonly prepared using this dry-heat cooking method. Steaming: Steaming helps preserve the natural moisture in seafood and is a good fit for delicate seafood that may not stand up to more aggressive cooking techniques. Use the moist-heat cooking method for shellfish, like clams and mussels, or crustaceans.

- **Grilling:**

Grilling is another dry-heat cooking method and one that often leads to sticking. Coating your grill grates with high–smoke point oil can help prevent this. Most fish can cook directly over the grates on a grill but can easily fall apart, so use care when flipping or turning. Meat Thermometer: A meat thermometer is the most accurate way to tell when fish is finished cooking. For most fish, cooking to 140 to 145ºF is a safe level that doesn't sacrifice the texture or flavor of the prepared dish. If you don't have a meat thermometer, look for an opaque color and firm, flaky texture to determine when your fish is well cooked.

Tips for Flavoring Fish

I often hear people comment on the lack of flavor in fish or the overly "fishy" taste. Neither bodes well for convincing them to include seafood more often.

Here are my top tips for flavoring fish:

- **Know your ingredients**

Understand the difference between fish, mollusks, and crustaceans to choose ingredients or cooking methods that will yield the best results. Think of your seafood selections in terms of texture (delicate, medium, or firm) and flavor (mild, moderate, or full), especially when looking for recipe substitutions.

- **Marination**

When marinating a fillet, make sure not to let it sit too long if it contains acidic flavors from citrus or vinegar sources, as this can cook the seafood. Using a milder marinade for a shorter amount of time is recommended. It's best to marinate fish for 30 minutes to 2 hours in the refrigerator.

Ensure you season both sides of the fish, not just the top. It will taste better this way and ensure that every bite is super flavorful.

- **Sautéing**

When sautéing fish, make sure the oil in the pan is hot enough before adding the fish. It will create a sear and prevent the fish from sticking to the pan.

For most fish cooked in a pan, cook it 70 percent on one side before gently flipping and lowering the heat. At this point, add herbs and aromatics to the pan and baste the fish with its drippings. The first side will be your presentation side.

- **Don't overcook it!**

Fish should always be juicy and tender, not dry and tough. It ought to easily separate using a fork. Give 5 minutes of rest before serving after you remove it from the pan or oven. It allows the fish to retain moisture and finish cooking while resting.

- **Incorporate acids and seasonings**

Acidic components (citrus, vinegar, wine, or pickled ingredients) and seasonings (herbs and spices) liven up your cooking. The more savory a dish, the more it needs something to perk it up. Acid is one of the basic tastes, so it takes priority for me, but adding seasonings takes a dish from good to great.

- **Choose sides that complement but don't compete**

Finally, keep your entrée as the star of the show by choosing side dishes that play a supporting role. A pescatarian menu should feature many vegetables, greens, and grains, but too much variety can be overwhelming.

- **Use salt**

Highly processed foods and restaurant recipes have left us wary of sodium. But most ingredients for home cooking are naturally low in sodium. Salt enhances other ingredients in your finished dishes.

4-Week Meal Plan

Week 1	Breakfast	Lunch	Snack	Dinner	Dessert
1	Creamy Cinnamon Oatmeal	Crispy Cod with Asparagus + Basil Guacamole	Roasted Broccoli	Red Beans & Rice	Melon-Lime Sorbet
2	Egg and Salmon Stuffed Avocado	Cauliflower Rice + Lentil with Paprika	Sweet Potato Fries	Roasted Chickpeas	Lemon Curd
3	Peach Muesli	Whole-Wheat Flatbread + Shrimp Ginger Soup	Crispy Baked Cauliflower	Tempeh with Fried Rice	Coconut-Quinoa Pudding
4	Spinach-Blueberry Smoothie	Brown Rice Stir Fry + Avocado and Quinoa Salad	Apple Snack	Quinoa Stuffed Sweet Potato	Easy Mango Sorbet
5	Egg White Omelet	Teriyaki Stir Fry+ Cobb salad	Fresh Pea Hummus	Succotash	Grilled Peaches
6	Peanut Butter Pancakes	Rustic Pasta	Tuna Stuffed Peppers	Rice with Shrimp	Peach Popsicles
7	Creamy Oats with Peach	Spinach and Mushroom Pasta	Salmon Pâté	Tomato and Chickpea Salad	Raspberry S'mores

Week 2	Breakfast	Lunch	Snack	Dinner	Dessert
1	Coconut-Mango Smoothie	Navy Bean Broccoli Toss + Mexican salsa	Fresh Pea Hummus	Quinoa Stuffed Sweet Potato	Chocolate Hummus
2	Breakfast Avocado Toast	Cajun Catfish and Shrimp + Basil Guacamole	Salmon Pâté	Lentil Quesadillas	Coconut-Quinoa Pudding
3	Egg White Omelet	Spinach and Mushroom Pasta	Tuna Stuffed Peppers	Tahini Falafels	Melon-Lime Sorbet
4	Spicy Tofu Tacos	Pecan Wild Rice + Carrot soup	Apple Snack	Tempeh with Fried Rice	Lemon Curd
5	Creamy Cinnamon Oatmeal	Whole-Wheat Flatbread + White Bean Stew with Cauliflower	Roasted Broccoli	Nutty Scallops	Easy Mango Sorbet
6	Peanut Butter Pancakes	Cauliflower rice + Sun-dried Tomato Snapper	Potted Salmon	Cauliflower Steaks	Raspberry S'mores
7	Egg and Salmon Stuffed Avocado	Shrimp with Pasta	Spicy Edamame	Roasted Chickpeas	Peach Popsicles

Week 3	Breakfast	Lunch	Snack	Dinner	Dessert
1	Egg White Omelet	Rustic pasta + Avocado and Quinoa Salad	Sweet Potato Fries	Succotash	Raspberry S'mores
2	Peach Muesli	Spaghetti with Radicchio+ Cobb Salad	Salmon Pâté	Brown Rice Stir Fry	Lemon Curd
3	Egg and Salmon Stuffed Avocado	Rice with Shrimp + Basil Guacamole	Crispy Baked Cauliflower	Potato and Salmon Soup	Baked Pears

4	Spicy Tofu Tacos	Red pepper pasta	Roasted Broccoli	Tomato and Crab Salad	Coconut-Quinoa Pudding
5	Spinach-Blueberry Smoothie	Tuna melts + Mexican salsa	Edamame Hummus	Lentil Potato Salad	Melon-Lime Sorbet
6	Creamy Cinnamon Oatmeal	Crispy Cod with Asparagus	Apple Snack	Mussels in Coconut Milk	No-Bake Cookie Dough
7	Coconut-Mango Smoothie	Tempeh with Fried Rice	Tuna Stuffed Peppers	Whitefish Soup	Peach Popsicles

Week 4	Breakfast	Lunch	Snack	Dinner	Dessert
1	Peach Muesli	Cauliflower Steaks + Baked salmon	Salmon Pâté	Cantaloupe Cold soup	Coconut-Quinoa Pudding
2	Creamy Oats with Peach	Red Beans & Rice	Roasted Broccoli	Chickpea-Stuffed Sweet Potatoes	Chocolate Hummus
3	Egg and Salmon Stuffed Avocado	Teriyaki Stir Fry	Apple Snack	Avocado and Quinoa Salad	No-Bake Cookie Dough
4	Spicy Tofu Tacos	Avocado and Quinoa Salad	Potted Salmon	Garlic Alfredo Pasta	Peach Popsicles
5	Coconut-Mango Smoothie	Spinach and Mushroom Pasta	Tuna Stuffed Peppers	Crispy Cod with Asparagus	Grilled Peaches
6	Creamy Cinnamon Oatmeal	Cauliflower Rice + Lentil potato salad	Sweet Potato Fries	Tomato and Chickpea Salad	Melon-Lime Sorbet
7	Peanut Butter Pancakes	Tomato and Chickpea Salad	Roasted Brussels sprouts	Quinoa–Sweet Potato Stew	Easy Mango Sorbet

CHAPTER 3

Breakfast And Brunch Recipes

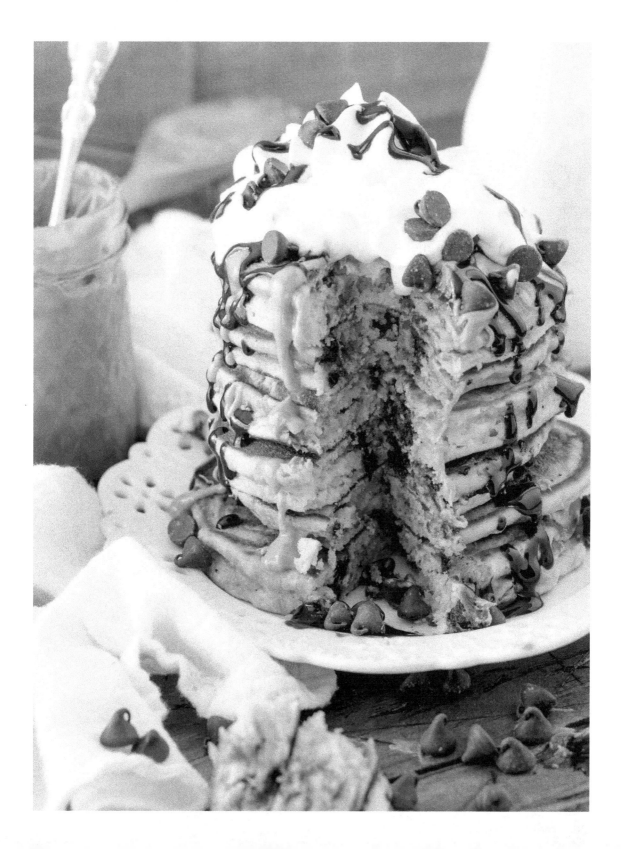

Creamy Cinnamon Oatmeal

Prep time: 5 minutes, cook time: 25 minutes; Serves 5

Ingredients:
- 1 apple, peeled, cored, and chopped
- 1 tablespoon ground cinnamon, plus more for serving
- 1 teaspoon nutmeg
- 2 teaspoons vanilla extract
- 1 cup steel-cut oats
- ½ cup cinnamon applesauce
- 3 cups 1% milk
- 6 ounces 2% vanilla Greek yogurt
- ½ cup walnuts, crushed

Instructions:
1. Boil the milk in a saucepan over medium heat
2. Then reduce to a simmer and add the apple, cinnamon, nutmeg, vanilla, oats, and applesauce.
3. Cover and cook for about seven minutes, stirring occasionally.
4. Turn off the heat, keeping the oats covered for another 3 minutes.
5. To serve, portion the oats into individual bowls and add a few spoonfuls of Greek yogurt to each bowl. Stir it in until creamy and smooth.
6. Sprinkle each serving with about 2 tablespoons walnuts and a dash of cinnamon.
7. Serve warm.

Nutrition Facts Per Serving

Calories 275, Total Fat 8g, Saturated Fat 3g, Total Carbs 35g, Protein 16g, Sugar:24g, Fiber:6g, Sodium 128mg, Omega-3 Fat: 926mg; Cholesterol: 16mg

Spinach-Blueberry Smoothie

Prep time: 5 minutes; Serves 2

Ingredients:
- 2 cups roughly chopped fresh spinach
- 1 cup blueberries
- 1 cup unsweetened vanilla almond milk
- ½ cup plain low-fat Greek yogurt
- ¼ cup rolled oats

Instructions:
1. In a blender, blend the spinach, blueberries, almond milk, yogurt, and oats until smooth.
2. Pour into 2 glasses and serve immediately.
3. Enjoy

Nutrition Facts Per Serving

Calories 118, Total Fat 3g, Saturated Fat 1g, Total Carbs 17g, Protein 8g, Fiber:3g, Sodium:124mg

Peanut Butter Pancakes

Prep time: 10 minutes, cook time: 15 minutes; Serves 4

Ingredients:

- 1½ cups whole-wheat flour
- 1 tablespoon baking powder
- ½ teaspoon salt
- 1½ cups unsweetened vanilla almond
- milk
- 1 egg
- 3 tablespoons peanut butter
- 1 tablespoon olive oil

Instructions:

1. In a bowl, mix well the flour, baking powder, and salt.
2. In another bowl, whisk together the almond milk, egg, and peanut butter.
3. Combine the flour and milk mixtures and stir well until the batter is smooth.
4. Heat the olive oil over medium heat in a skillet and pour about ¼ cup of batter into the skillet for each pancake.
5. Cook until it browns on both sides of the pancake.
6. Repeat with the remaining batter.
7. Serve warm with your choice of topping.

Nutrition Facts Per Serving

Calories 284, Total Fat 11g, Saturated Fat 2g, Total Carbs 36g, Protein 12g, Fiber:7g, Sodium465 mg

Egg and Salmon Stuffed Avocado

Prep time: 5 minutes, cook time: 22 minutes; Serves 6

Ingredients:

- 3 ripe avocados
- 6 thinly sliced pieces smoked salmon
- 6 eggs
- Freshly ground black pepper to taste
- Salt to taste

Instructions:

1. Preheat the oven to 450°F, meanwhile, line a baking sheet with parchment paper.
2. Cut each avocado in half and take the pit out. Take out some avocado from each center, making more room for the filling.
3. Place the avocado halves on the prepared baking sheet. Gently layer each avocado half with a piece of salmon, pressing the salmon, so there is still a depression where the pit used to be.
4. In a small bowl, crack one egg.
5. Transfer the yolk and as much white as fits to the center of the avocado half.
6. Repeat with the remaining 5 eggs and avocado halves. Sprinkle with black pepper to taste.
7. Bake until the egg sets.
8. Add a few shakes of everything-bagel seasoning to each avocado and devour!

Nutrition Facts Per Serving

Calories 257, Total Fat 20g, Saturated Fat 4 g, Total Carbs 8g, Protein 15g, Sugar: 6g, Fiber: 5g, Sodium: 402mg Omega-3 Fat: 258mg Cholesterol: 173mg

Coconut-Mango Smoothie

Prep time: 5 minutes; Serves 2

Ingredients:
- 1 cup of ice cubes
- 1 cup frozen mango chunks
- 1 cup frozen pineapple chunks
- 1 cup unsweetened coconut milk
- 2 tablespoons unsweetened coconut flakes
- 1 tablespoon chia seeds (optional)

Instructions:
1. In a blender, put the ice, mango, pineapple, and coconut milk or almond milk then pulse until smooth.
2. Serve in two glasses with a sprinkle of coconut flakes and chia seeds.

Nutrition Facts Per Serving

Calories 263, Total Fat10g, Saturated Fat, Total Carbs 41g, Protein2g, and Sugar: 36g, Sodium: 88mg

Egg White Omelet

Prep time: 10 minutes, cook time: 10 minutes; Serves 2

Ingredients:
- 1 teaspoon olive oil
- ½ cup loosely packed spinach leaves
- ¼ cup diced red onion
- 2 garlic cloves, minced
- ¼ cup diced tomatoes
- 2 eggs
- 4 egg whites
- 2 tablespoons almond milk
- 2 tablespoons crumbled feta cheese

Instructions:
1. Heat the olive oil in a nonstick skillet over medium heat. Add the spinach, onion, and garlic, and cook for 3 minutes.
2. Add the tomatoes and cook for 2 minutes more, stirring occasionally.
3. In a small bowl, whisk together the eggs, egg whites, and almond milk.
4. Add the egg mixture to the skillet, tilting the pan to coat the spinach mixture with the eggs.
5. Cook for 3 minutes until the eggs almost set, stirring gently, so the eggs cook evenly and tilting the pan to let the softer parts of the egg mixture flow to the edges to cook.
6. Scatter the cheese over the top, and continue to cook for 2 minutes until the eggs are set but still moist.
7. Carefully fold the omelet in half, then cut into two pieces and serve.

Nutrition Facts Per Serving

Calories 158, Total Fat 9g, Total Carbs 5g, Protein 15g, Fiber:1g, Sodium: 241mg

Spicy Tofu Tacos

Prep time: 10 minutes, cook time: 10 minutes; Serves 4

Ingredients:

- 1 tablespoon olive oil
- ½ sweet onion, finely chopped
- 1 jalapeño, seeded and finely chopped
- 1 pound extra-firm tofu, diced
- Sea salt and black pepper, for
seasoning
- 4 hard corn taco shells, warmed
- 1 cup store-bought salsa, for topping
- 1 cup shredded low-fat Cheddar cheese, for topping

Instructions:

1. In a skillet, heat the olive oil over medium-high heat.
2. Sauté the onion and jalapeño pepper until softened, about 3 minutes.
3. Stir in the tofu and then season with salt and pepper.
4. Sauté until golden brown, about 7 minutes (It is okay if the tofu breaks up.)
5. Divide the tofu mixture between the taco shells.
6. Top each taco with a portion of the salsa and the cheese before serving.

Nutrition Facts Per Serving

Calories 331, Total Fat 21g, Saturated Fat 6g, Total Carbs17g, Protein 23g, Fiber:3g, Sodium:510 mg

Creamy Oats with Peach

Prep time: 5 minutes, cook time: 10 minutes; Serves 2

Ingredients:

- 1 cup uncooked rolled oats
- 1½ cups plain, low-fat kefir
- ¼ cup chopped pecans
- 2 tablespoons hemp hearts
- 1 teaspoon ground cinnamon
- ½ teaspoon vanilla extract
- 1½ cups of diced peaches
- 2 teaspoons honey

Instructions:

1. Divide the oats, kefir, pecans, hemp hearts, cinnamon, and vanilla between two mason jars or food storage containers. Stir gently to combine, and then top with the diced peaches.
2. Seal and refrigerate to chill overnight.
3. When ready to serve, drizzle the honey over the top.
4. Stir to combine before eating.

Nutrition Facts Per Serving

Calories440, Total Fat 25g, Saturated Fat 3g, Total Carbs 54g, Protein 19g, Sugar:23g, Fiber:9g, Sodium:95 mg

Breakfast Avocado Toast

Prep time: 10 minutes, cook time: 10 minutes; Serves 1

Ingredients:
- 1 whole-wheat English muffin, halved
- ½ ripe avocado cut into ¼-inch cubes
- 3 fresh basil leaves, chopped
- ½ a cup halved cherry tomatoes
- 1-ounce fresh mozzarella pearls halved
- 2 teaspoons balsamic glaze

Instructions:
1. Lightly toast the English muffin.
2. Mash the avocado with a spoon and then scoop the mash onto the two halves of the English muffin.
3. Layer the fresh basil on top of the avocado.
4. Arrange the cherry tomatoes and mozzarella pearls, flat-side down, on top of the basil.
5. Drizzle each half with the balsamic glaze and serve immediately.

Nutrition Facts Per Serving

Calories350, Total Fat16g, Saturated Fat4.5g, Total Carbs39g, Protein 15g, Sugar: 0g, Fiber: 10g, Sodium: 420mg

Peach Muesli

Prep time: 10 minutes, Chill time: 12 Hours; Serves 4

Ingredients:
- 2 cups plain low-fat Greek yogurt
- 2 cups gluten-free rolled oats
- ½ cup unsweetened shredded coconut
- 2 tablespoons maple syrup
- 2 ripe peaches, pitted and roughly chopped

Instructions:
1. Preheat the oven to 250°F and spread the shredded coconut on a baking sheet.
2. Toast the coconut in the oven until golden brown and fragrant, occasionally stirring, about 15 minutes.
3. In a large resealable container, stir together the yogurt, oats, coconut, and maple syrup.
4. Seal the container and put it in the refrigerator overnight.
5. Stir in the peaches in the morning and serve. Flavor Boost for a deeper, richer flavor, try toasting the shredded coconut before stirring it into this simple breakfast.

Nutrition Facts Per Serving

Calories 286, Total Fat11g, Saturated Fat 7g, Total Carbs 31g, Protein 15g, Fiber: 5g, Sodium:56mg

CHAPTER 4

Fish and Seafood Recipes

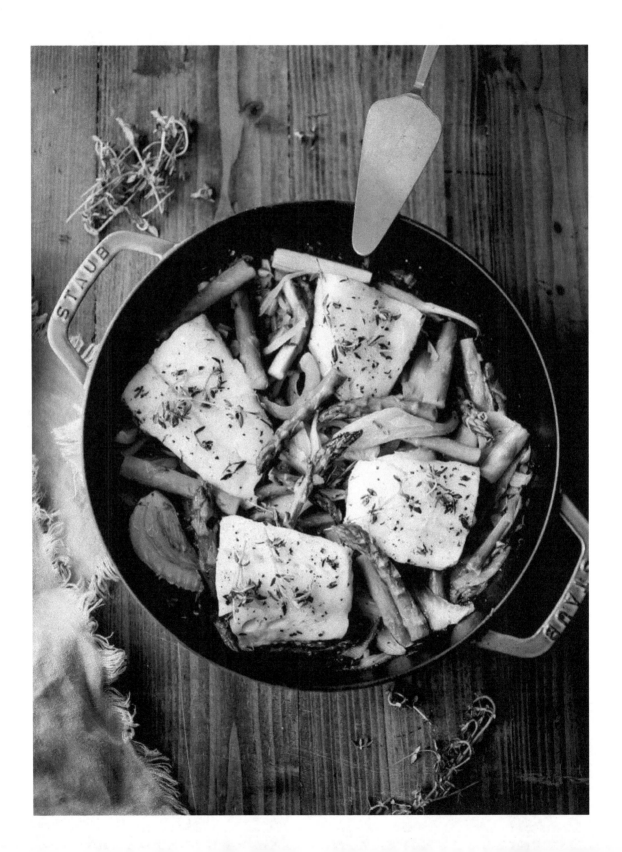

Crispy Cod with Asparagus

Prep time: 5 minutes, cook time: 15 minutes; Serves 4

Ingredients:
- 2 teaspoons Old Bay Seasoning
- ½ cup whole-wheat panko bread crumbs
- 1 pound asparagus, trimmed
- 1½ tablespoons olive oil, divided
- 4 (5-ounce) cod fillets
- Juice of 1 lemon

Instructions:
1. Preheat the oven to 375°F then line a rimmed baking sheet with aluminum foil or parchment paper. Mix the Old Bay Seasoning and bread crumbs in a bowl and set aside.
2. Spread the asparagus on the prepared baking sheet.
3. Drizzle 1 tablespoon of olive oil over the asparagus using your hands or tongs; gently toss the asparagus until evenly coated with oil.
4. Sprinkle half of the bread crumb mixture over the asparagus, reserving the rest for the fish.
5. Pat the cod fillets dry and brush them lightly with the remaining ½ tablespoon of olive oil. Drizzle the lemon juice over the fillets.
6. Dip each fillet in the seasoned bread crumbs and then place it on the same baking sheet as the asparagus.
7. Bake until the fish is no longer translucent and flakes easily, 10 to 15 minutes. Serve the cod with the asparagus immediately.

Nutrition Facts Per Serving

Calories 236, Total Fat 8g, Saturated Fat 1g, Total Carbs 14g, Protein 29g, Sugar:3g, Fiber:3g, Sodium:511mg

Fish–Stuffed Avocados

Prep time: 15 minutes; Serves 4

Ingredients:
- 4 avocados, pitted
- ½ pound crabmeat
- ½ pound cooked shrimp, peeled, deveined and roughly chopped
- 1 red bell pepper, seeded and finely chopped
- 1 scallion, sliced
- Sea salt, and freshly ground black pepper for seasoning

Instructions:
1. Scoop out the center of the avocados, leaving a ½-inch layer of fruit in each half.
2. Transfer the scooped-out portion to a large bowl and set the avocado halves aside.
3. Add the crabmeat, shrimp, bell pepper, and scallion to the bowl and mix well.
4. Season the filling with salt and pepper.
5. Spoon the seafood filling into the avocado halves and serve immediately.

Nutrition Facts Per Serving

Calories 418, Total Fat 28g, Saturated Fat 4g, Total Carbs 19g, Protein 23g, Fiber:12g, Sodium:466mg

Cajun Catfish and Shrimp

Prep time: 10 minutes, cook time: 30 minutes; Serves 4

Ingredients:

- 4 (4-ounce) catfish fillets, cut into two pieces each
- ½ pound shrimp, peeled and deveined
- 1 tablespoon Cajun seasoning
- 4 russet potatoes cut into eighths
- 2 ears of corn cut into four pieces
- ½ cup of water
- Sea salt, and freshly ground black pepper for seasoning

Instructions:

1. Preheat the oven to 400°F
2. Cut 4 pieces of aluminum foil, each 12 inches square with the edges turned up to form a rough bowl and set aside.
3. In a medium bowl, toss the catfish, shrimp, and Cajun seasoning together until well combined. Divide the potatoes and corn between the foil pieces and top with the catfish and shrimp.
4. Drizzle the fish and vegetables with water and lightly season with salt and pepper.
5. Fold the foil up to form tightly sealed packets and put them on a baking sheet.
6. Bake until the fish flakes when pressed with a fork and the vegetables are tender, for about half an hour.

Nutrition Facts Per Serving

Calories 349, Total Fat 7g, Saturated Fat 1g, Total Carbs 48g, Protein 28g, Fiber:7g, Sodium:219mg

Coconut Crab Cakes

Prep time: 10 minutes, chill time: 1 hour Cook time: 10 minutes; Serves 4

Ingredients:

- 1 pound canned crabmeat, drained
- ¼ cup coconut flour
- 1 scallion, finely chopped
- 1 egg, beaten
- ½ teaspoon minced garlic
- Juice and zest of ½ a lemon
- Sea salt, and freshly ground black pepper for seasoning
- 2 tablespoons olive oil

Instructions:

1. In a medium bowl, mix the crabmeat, coconut flour, scallion, egg, garlic, lemon juice, and lemon zest.
2. Season the crab mixture with salt and pepper.
3. Divide the crab mixture into eight cakes about 1-inch thick.
4. Chill the crab cakes, covered, in the refrigerator for 1 hour to firm them up.
5. In a large skillet, heat the olive oil over medium-high heat.
6. Pan sear the crab cakes until they are golden on both sides, turning once, about 5 minutes per side.

Nutrition Facts Per Serving

Calories 256, Total Fat12g, Saturated Fat 3g, Total Carbs 11g, Protein 27g, Fiber:6g, Sodium:393mg

Mussels in Coconut Milk

Prep time: 10 minutes, cook time: 15 minutes; Serves 4

Ingredients:

- 2 tablespoons olive oil
- ½ sweet onion, finely chopped
- 1 tablespoon minced garlic
- 2 teaspoons grated fresh ginger
- 1 tablespoon curry powder
- 1 cup of coconut milk
- 1½ pounds fresh mussels, scrubbed and debearded
- 2 tablespoons finely chopped cilantro

Instructions:

1. In a large skillet, heat the olive oil over medium-high heat and sauté the onion, garlic, and ginger until softened about 3 minutes.
2. Add the curry powder and toss to combine.
3. Stir in the coconut milk and bring to a boil.
4. Add the mussels, cover, and steam until the shells are open, about 8 minutes.
5. Remove any unopened shells and take the skillet off the heat.
6. Stir in the cilantro and serve.

Nutrition Facts Per Serving

Calories 263, Total Fat23g, Saturated Fat14g, Total Carbs 9g, Protein 9g, Fiber: 2g, Sodium: 172mg

Baked Salmon

Prep time: 10 minutes, cook time: 25 minutes; Serves 4

Ingredients:

- 4 (4-ounce) boneless, skinless salmon fillets
- Sea salt, and freshly ground black pepper for seasoning
- ½ cup of coconut milk
- 1 cup shredded unsweetened coconut
- 1 tablespoon olive oil
- 1 tablespoon finely chopped fresh cilantro

Instructions:

1. Preheat the oven to 400°F then line a baking sheet with parchment paper and set aside.
2. Pat, the salmon, fillets dry with paper towels and lightly season them with salt and pepper.
3. Pour the coconut milk into a medium bowl and the shredded coconut in another medium bowl.
4. Dredge the fillets in the coconut milk and then press the fish into the shredded coconut, so both sides of each piece are well coated.
5. Put the fillets on the prepared baking sheet and drizzle with olive oil.
6. Bake the salmon until the topping is golden and the fish flakes easily with a fork, 12 to 15 minutes.
7. Serve topped with cilantro.

Nutrition Facts Per Serving

Calories 370, Total Fat 29g, Saturated Fat 15g, Total Carbs 5g, Protein 23g, Fiber:3g, Sodium:132mg

Nutty Scallops

Prep time: 10 minutes, cook time: 10 minutes; Serves 4

Ingredients:
- 1 pound sea scallops, cleaned
- Sea salt and freshly ground black pepper for seasoning
- 1 cup crushed pistachios
- 2 tablespoons extra-virgin olive oil
- 2 tablespoons butter
- Juice of 1 lime

Instructions:
1. Pat the scallops dry with a paper towel and season them lightly on all sides with salt and pepper. Place the pistachios in a large bowl and dredge the scallops in the crushed nuts, making sure to coat all sides.
2. In a large skillet, heat the olive oil over high heat.
3. Sear the scallops until they are golden brown, about 2 minutes, and then turn them over.
4. Add the butter to the skillet and continue cooking the scallops 3 minutes more.
5. Serve immediately with a squeeze of lime juice.

Nutrition Facts Per Serving
Calories 351, Total Fat 24g, Saturated Fat 6g, Total Carbs 10g, Protein 24g, Fiber:2g, Sodium:247mg

Garlic Shrimp with Arugula Pesto

Prep time: 20 minutes, Cook time: 5 minutes, Serves 2

Ingredients:
- 3 cups lightly packed arugula
- ½ cup lightly packed basil leaves
- ¼ cup walnuts
- 3 tablespoons olive oil
- 3 medium garlic cloves
- 2 tablespoons grated Parmesan cheese
- 1 tablespoon freshly squeezed lemon
- juice
- Salt and freshly ground black pepper, to taste
- 1 (10-ounce / 283-g) package zucchini noodles
- 8 ounces (227 g) cooked, shelled shrimp
- 2 Roma tomatoes, diced

Instructions:
1. Process the arugula, basil, walnuts, olive oil, garlic, Parmesan cheese, and lemon juice in a food processor until smooth, scraping down the sides as needed. Season with salt and pepper to taste.
2. Heat a skillet over medium heat. Add the pesto, zucchini noodles, and cooked shrimp. Toss to combine the sauce over the noodles and shrimp, and cook until heated through.
3. Taste and season with more salt and pepper as needed. Serve topped with the diced tomatoes.

Nutrition Facts Per Serving
calories: 435, fat: 30.2g, protein: 33.0g, carbs: 15.1g, fiber: 5.0g, sodium: 413mg

Tuna Melts

Prep time: 5 minutes, cook time: 5 minutes; Serves 4

Ingredients:

- 4 thick slices of rye or whole-wheat bread
- 2 (5-ounce) cans tuna, drained
- ¼ cup cottage cheese
- ⅓ cup of chopped sun-dried tomatoes
- 1 apple, peeled and thinly sliced
- 4 slices sharp Cheddar cheese

Instructions:

1. Preheat the oven to 400°F then line a baking sheet with aluminum foil.
2. Lightly toast the bread and then place it on the baking sheet.
3. In a large bowl, mix the tuna, cottage cheese, and sun-dried tomatoes.
4. Build the sandwiches by layering the apples on the bottom and topping with the tuna mixture. Place the cheese on top, then broil for 5 minutes, or until the cheese is fully melted.
5. Serve hot.

Nutrition Facts Per Serving

Calories 360, Total Fat 13g, Saturated Fat 7g, Total Carbs 25g, Protein 32g, Sugar:8g, Fiber:3g, Sodium:750mg

Dill Chutney Salmon

Prep time: 5 minutes, Cook time: 3 minutes, Serves 2

Ingredients:

Chutney:

- ¼ cup fresh dill
- ¼ cup extra virgin olive oil
- Juice from ½ lemon
- Sea salt, to taste

Fish:

- 2 cups water
- 2 salmon fillets
- Juice from ½ lemon
- ¼ teaspoon paprika
- Salt and freshly ground pepper to taste

Instructions:

1. Pulse all the chutney ingredients in a food processor until creamy. Set aside.
2. Add the water and steamer basket to the Instant Pot. Place salmon fillets, skin-side down, on the steamer basket. Drizzle the lemon juice over salmon and sprinkle with the paprika.
3. Secure the lid. Select the Manual mode and set the cooking time for 3 minutes at High Pressure.
4. Once cooking is complete, do a quick pressure release. Carefully open the lid.
5. Season the fillets with pepper and salt to taste. Serve topped with the dill chutney.

Nutrition Facts Per Serving

calories: 636, fat: 41.1g, protein: 65.3g, carbs: 1.9g, fiber: 0.2g, sodium: 477mg

Sun-dried Tomato Snapper

Prep time: 10 minutes, cook time: 20 minutes; Serves 4

Ingredients:

- 1 sweet onion, cut into ¼-inch slices
- 4 (5-ounce) snapper fillets
- Freshly ground black pepper, for seasoning
- ¼ cup sun-dried tomato pesto
- 2 tablespoons finely chopped fresh basil
- For the sun-dried tomato pesto
- 1 cup sun-dried tomatoes
- ½ cup basil
- ¼ cup Parmesan cheese
- ¼ cup olive oil
- 4 garlic cloves

Instructions:

1. Preheat the oven to 400°F then line a baking dish with parchment paper and arrange the onion slices on the bottom.
2. Pat the snapper fillets dry with a paper towel and season them lightly with pepper.
3. Place the fillets on the onions and spread one tablespoon of tomato pesto on each fillet.
4. Bake until the fish flakes easily with a fork, 12 to 15 minutes.
5. Serve topped with basil.
6. For the sun-dried tomato pesto
7. Pulse the sun-dried tomatoes, basil, Parmesan cheese, olive oil, and garlic cloves until thick paste forms.

Nutrition Facts Per Serving

Calories 199, Total Fat 3g, Saturated Fat 0g, Total Carbs 3g, Protein 36g, Fiber:1g, Sodium:119mg

Slow Cooker Salmon in Foil

Prep time: 5 minutes, Cook time: 2 hours, Serves 2

Ingredients:

- 2 (6-ounce / 170-g) salmon fillets
- 1 tablespoon olive oil
- 2 cloves garlic, minced
- ½ tablespoon lime juice
- 1 teaspoon finely chopped fresh parsley
- ¼ teaspoon black pepper

Instructions:

1. Spread a length of foil onto a work surface and place the salmon fillets in the middle.
2. Mix together the olive oil, garlic, lime juice, parsley, and black pepper in a small bowl. Brush the mixture over the fillets. Fold the foil over and crimp the sides to make a packet.
3. Place the packet into the slow cooker, cover, and cook on High for 2 hours, or until the fish flakes easily with a fork.
4. Serve hot.

Nutrition Facts Per Serving

calories: 446, fat: 20.7g, protein: 65.4g, carbs: 1.5g, fiber: 0.2g, sodium: 240mg

Hazelnut Crusted Sea Bass

Prep time: 10 minutes, Cook time: 15 minutes, Serves 2

Ingredients:

- 2 tablespoons almond butter
- 2 sea bass fillets
- ⅓ cup roasted hazelnuts
- A pinch of cayenne pepper

Instructions:

1. Preheat the oven to 425°F (220°C). Line a baking dish with waxed paper.
2. Brush the almond butter over the fillets.
3. Pulse the hazelnuts and cayenne in a food processor. Coat the sea bass with the hazelnut mixture, then transfer to the baking dish.
4. Bake in the preheated oven for about 15 minutes. Cool for 5 minutes before serving.

Nutrition Facts Per Serving

calories: 468, fat: 30.8g, protein: 40.0g, carbs: 8.8g, fiber: 4.1g, sodium: 90mg

Lemon Rosemary Roasted Branzino

Prep time: 15 minutes, Cook time: 30 minutes, Serves 2

Ingredients:

- 4 tablespoons extra-virgin olive oil, divided
- 2 (8-ounce / 227-g) branzino fillets, preferably at least 1 inch thick
- 1 garlic clove, minced
- 1 bunch scallions (white part only), thinly sliced
- 10 to 12 small cherry tomatoes, halved
- 1 large carrot, cut into ¼-inch rounds
- ½ cup dry white wine
- 2 tablespoons paprika
- 2 teaspoons kosher salt
- ½ tablespoon ground chili pepper
- 2 rosemary sprigs or 1 tablespoon dried rosemary
- 1 small lemon, thinly sliced
- ½ cup sliced pitted kalamata olives

Instructions:

1. Heat a large ovenproof skillet over high heat until hot, about 2 minutes. Add 1 tablespoon of olive oil and heat for 10 to 15 seconds until it shimmers.
2. Add the branzino fillets, skin-side up, and sear for 2 minutes. Flip the fillets and cook for an additional 2 minutes. Set aside.
3. Swirl 2 tablespoons of olive oil around the skillet to coat evenly.
4. Add the garlic, scallions, tomatoes, and carrot, and sauté for 5 minutes, or until softened.
5. Add the wine, stirring until all ingredients are well combined. Carefully place the fish over the sauce.
6. Preheat the oven to 450°F (235°C).
7. Brush the fillets with the remaining 1 tablespoon of olive oil and season with paprika, salt, and chili pepper. Top each fillet with a rosemary sprig and lemon slices. Scatter the olives over fish and around the skillet.
8. Roast for about 10 minutes until the lemon slices are browned. Serve hot.

Nutrition Facts Per Serving

calories: 724, fat: 43.0g, protein: 57.7g, carbs: 25.0g, fiber: 10.0g, sodium: 2950mg

Grilled Lemon Pesto Salmon

Prep time: 5 minutes, Cook time: 6 to 10 minutes, Serves 2

Ingredients:
- 10 ounces (283 g) salmon fillet (1 large piece or 2 smaller ones)
- Salt and freshly ground black pepper, to taste
- 2 tablespoons prepared pesto sauce
- 1 large fresh lemon, sliced
- Cooking spray

Instructions:
1. Preheat the grill to medium-high heat. Spray the grill grates with cooking spray.
2. Season the salmon with salt and black pepper. Spread the pesto sauce on top.
3. Make a bed of fresh lemon slices about the same size as the salmon fillet on the hot grill, and place the salmon on top of the lemon slices. Put any additional lemon slices on top of the salmon.
4. Grill the salmon for 6 to 10 minutes, or until the fish is opaque and flakes apart easily.
5. Serve hot.

Nutrition Facts Per Serving

calories: 316, fat: 21.1g, protein: 29.0g, carbs: 1.0g, fiber: 0g, sodium: 175mg

Roasted Trout Stuffed with Veggies

Prep time: 10 minutes, Cook time: 25 minutes, Serves 2

Ingredients:
- 2 (8-ounce / 227-g) whole trout fillets, dressed (cleaned but with bones and skin intact)
- 1 tablespoon extra-virgin olive oil
- ¼ teaspoon salt
- ⅛ teaspoon freshly ground black pepper
- 1 small onion, thinly sliced
- ½ red bell pepper, seeded and thinly sliced
- 1 poblano pepper, seeded and thinly sliced
- 2 or 3 shiitake mushrooms, sliced
- 1 lemon, sliced
- Nonstick cooking spray

Instructions:
1. Preheat the oven to 425ºF (220ºC). Spray a baking sheet with nonstick cooking spray.
2. Rub both trout fillets, inside and out, with the olive oil. Season with salt and pepper.
3. Mix together the onion, bell pepper, poblano pepper, and mushrooms in a large bowl. Stuff half of this mixture into the cavity of each fillet. Top the mixture with 2 or 3 lemon slices inside each fillet.
4. Place the fish on the prepared baking sheet side by side. Roast in the preheated oven for 25 minutes, or until the fish is cooked through and the vegetables are tender.
5. Remove from the oven and serve on a plate.

Nutrition Facts Per Serving

calories: 453, fat: 22.1g, protein: 49.0g, carbs: 13.8g, fiber: 3.0g, sodium: 356mg

Easy Tomato Tuna Melts

Prep time: 5 minutes, Cook time: 3 to 4 minutes, Serves 2

Ingredients:
- 1 (5-ounce / 142-g) can chunk light tuna packed in water, drained
- 2 tablespoons plain Greek yogurt
- 2 tablespoons finely chopped celery
- 1 tablespoon finely chopped red onion
- 2 teaspoons freshly squeezed lemon juice
- Pinch cayenne pepper
- 1 large tomato, cut into ¾-inch-thick rounds
- ½ cup shredded Cheddar cheese

Instructions:
1. Preheat the broiler to High.
2. Stir together the tuna, yogurt, celery, red onion, lemon juice, and cayenne pepper in a medium bowl.
3. Place the tomato rounds on a baking sheet. Top each with some tuna salad and Cheddar cheese.
4. Broil for 3 to 4 minutes until the cheese is melted and bubbly. Cool for 5 minutes before serving.

Nutrition Facts Per Serving

calories: 244, fat: 10.0g, protein: 30.1g, carbs: 6.9g, fiber: 1.0g, sodium: 445mg

Mackerel and Green Bean Salad

Prep time: 10 minutes, Cook time: 10 minutes, Serves 2

Ingredients:
- 2 cups green beans
- 1 tablespoon avocado oil
- 2 mackerel fillets
- 4 cups mixed salad greens
- 2 hard-boiled eggs, sliced
- 1 avocado, sliced
- 2 tablespoons lemon juice
- 2 tablespoons olive oil
- 1 teaspoon Dijon mustard
- Salt and black pepper, to taste

Instructions:
1. Cook the green beans in a medium saucepan of boiling water for about 3 minutes until crisp-tender. Drain and set aside.
2. Melt the avocado oil in a pan over medium heat. Add the mackerel fillets and cook each side for 4 minutes.
3. Divide the greens between two salad bowls. Top with the mackerel, sliced egg, and avocado slices.
4. In another bowl, whisk together the lemon juice, olive oil, mustard, salt, and pepper, and drizzle over the salad. Add the cooked green beans and toss to combine, then serve.

Nutrition Facts Per Serving

calories: 737, fat: 57.3g, protein: 34.2g, carbs: 22.1g, fiber: 13.4g, sodium: 398mg

Shrimp and Pea Paella

Prep time: 20 minutes, Cook time: 60 minutes, Serves 2

Ingredients:

- 2 tablespoons olive oil
- 1 garlic clove, minced
- ½ large onion, minced
- 1 cup diced tomato
- ½ cup short-grain rice
- ½ teaspoon sweet paprika
- ½ cup dry white wine
- 1¼ cups low-sodium chicken stock
- 8 ounces (227 g) large raw shrimp
- 1 cup frozen peas
- ¼ cup jarred roasted red peppers, cut into strips
- Salt, to taste

Instructions:

Heat the olive oil in a large skillet over medium-high heat.
1. Add the garlic and onion and sauté for 3 minutes, or until the onion is softened.
2. Add the tomato, rice, and paprika and stir for 3 minutes to toast the rice.
3. Add the wine and chicken stock and stir to combine. Bring the mixture to a boil.
4. Cover and reduce the heat to medium-low, and simmer for 45 minutes, or until the rice is just about tender and most of the liquid has been absorbed.
5. Add the shrimp, peas, and roasted red peppers. Cover and cook for an additional 5 minutes. Season with salt to taste and serve.

Nutrition Facts Per Serving

calories: 646, fat: 27.1g, protein: 42.0g, carbs: 59.7g, fiber: 7.0g, sodium: 687mg

Steamed Trout with Lemon Herb Crust

Prep time: 10 minutes, Cook time: 15 minutes, Serves 2

Ingredients:

- 3 tablespoons olive oil
- 3 garlic cloves, chopped
- 2 tablespoons fresh lemon juice
- 1 tablespoon chopped fresh mint
- 1 tablespoon chopped fresh parsley
- ¼ teaspoon dried ground thyme
- 1 teaspoon sea salt
- 1 pound (454 g) fresh trout (2 pieces)
- 2 cups fish stock

Instructions:

1. Stir together the olive oil, garlic, lemon juice, mint, parsley, thyme, and salt in a small bowl. Brush the marinade onto the fish.
2. Insert a trivet in the Instant Pot. Pour in the fish stock and place the fish on the trivet.
3. Secure the lid. Select the Steam mode and set the cooking time for 15 minutes at High Pressure.
4. Once cooking is complete, do a quick pressure release. Carefully open the lid. Serve warm.

Nutrition Facts Per Serving

calories: 477, fat: 29.6g, protein: 51.7g, carbs: 3.6g, fiber: 0.2g, sodium: 2011mg

Baked Cod with Vegetables

Prep time: 15 minutes, Cook time: 25 minutes, Serves 2

Ingredients:

- 1 pound (454 g) thick cod fillet, cut into 4 even portions
- ¼ teaspoon onion powder (optional)
- ¼ teaspoon paprika
- 3 tablespoons extra-virgin olive oil
- 4 medium scallions
- ½ cup fresh chopped basil, divided
- 3 tablespoons minced garlic (optional)
- 2 teaspoons salt
- 2 teaspoons freshly ground black pepper
- ¼ teaspoon dry marjoram (optional)
- 6 sun-dried tomato slices
- ½ cup dry white wine
- ½ cup crumbled feta cheese
- 1 (15-ounce / 425-g) can oil-packed artichoke hearts, drained
- 1 lemon, sliced
- 1 cup pitted kalamata olives
- 1 teaspoon capers (optional)
- 4 small red potatoes, quartered

Instructions:

1. Preheat the oven to 375ºF (190ºC).
2. Season the fish with paprika and onion powder (if desired).
3. Heat an ovenproof skillet over medium heat and sear the top side of the cod for about 1 minute until golden. Set aside.
4. Heat the olive oil in the same skillet over medium heat. Add the scallions, ¼ cup of basil, garlic (if desired), salt, pepper, marjoram (if desired), tomato slices, and white wine and stir to combine. Bring to a boil and remove from heat.
5. Evenly spread the sauce on the bottom of skillet. Place the cod on top of the tomato basil sauce and scatter with feta cheese. Place the artichokes in the skillet and top with the lemon slices.
6. Scatter with the olives, capers (if desired), and the remaining ¼ cup of basil. Remove from the heat and transfer to the preheated oven. Bake for 15 to 20 minutes, or until it flakes easily with a fork.
7. Meanwhile, place the quartered potatoes on a baking sheet or wrapped in aluminum foil. Bake in the oven for 15 minutes until fork-tender.
8. Cool for 5 minutes before serving.

Nutrition Facts Per Serving

calories: 1168, fat: 60.0g, protein: 63.8g, carbs: 94.0g, fiber: 13.0g, sodium: 4620mg

Garlic-Butter Parmesan Salmon and Asparagus

Prep time: 10 minutes, Cook time: 15 minutes, Serves 2

Ingredients:

- 2 (6-ounce / 170-g) salmon fillets, skin on and patted dry
- Pink Himalayan salt
- Freshly ground black pepper, to taste
- 1 pound (454 g) fresh asparagus,
- ends snapped off
- 3 tablespoons almond butter
- 2 garlic cloves, minced
- ¼ cup grated Parmesan cheese

Instructions:

1. Preheat the oven to 400ºF (205ºC). Line a baking sheet with aluminum foil.

2. Season both sides of the salmon fillets with salt and pepper.
3. Put the salmon in the middle of the baking sheet and arrange the asparagus around the salmon.
4. Heat the almond butter in a small saucepan over medium heat.
5. Add the minced garlic and cook for about 3 minutes, or until the garlic just begins to brown.
6. Drizzle the garlic-butter sauce over the salmon and asparagus and scatter the Parmesan cheese on top.
7. Bake in the preheated oven for about 12 minutes, or until the salmon is cooked through and the asparagus is crisp-tender. You can switch the oven to broil at the end of cooking time for about 3 minutes to get a nice char on the asparagus.
8. Let cool for 5 minutes before serving.

Nutrition Facts Per Serving
calories: 435, fat: 26.1g, protein: 42.3g, carbs: 10.0g, fiber: 5.0g, sodium: 503mg

Lemony Trout with Caramelized Shallots

Prep time: 10 minutes, Cook time: 20 minutes, Serves 2

Ingredients:
Shallots:
- 1 teaspoon almond butter
- 2 shallots, thinly sliced
- Dash salt

Trout:
- 1 tablespoon plus 1 teaspoon almond butter, divided
- 2 (4-ounce / 113-g) trout fillets
- 3 tablespoons capers
- ¼ cup freshly squeezed lemon juice
- ¼ teaspoon salt
- Dash freshly ground black pepper
- 1 lemon, thinly sliced

Instructions:
Make the Shallots
1. In a large skillet over medium heat, cook the butter, shallots, and salt for 20 minutes, stirring every 5 minutes, or until the shallots are wilted and caramelized.

Make the Trout
2. Meanwhile, in another large skillet over medium heat, heat 1 teaspoon of almond butter.
3. Add the trout fillets and cook each side for 3 minutes, or until flaky. Transfer to a plate and set aside.
4. In the skillet used for the trout, stir in the capers, lemon juice, salt, and pepper, then bring to a simmer. Whisk in the remaining 1 tablespoon of almond butter. Spoon the sauce over the fish.
5. Garnish the fish with the lemon slices and caramelized shallots before serving.

Nutrition Facts Per Serving
calories: 344, fat: 18.4g, protein: 21.1g, carbs: 14.7g, fiber: 5.0g, sodium: 1090mg

Shrimp with Pasta

Prep time: 10 minutes, cook time: 20 minutes; Serves 4

Ingredients:

- ½ cup extra-virgin olive oil
- 5 rosemary sprigs
- 2 teaspoons fresh oregano
- 10 garlic cloves, peeled
- ¼ teaspoon red pepper flakes
- ¼ teaspoon salt
- ¼ teaspoon of freshly ground black

- pepper
- 1 lemon, halved then sliced, divided
- 1 small head broccoli
- 1 pound jumbo shrimp, peeled and deveined
- 12 ounces uncooked thin spaghetti

Instructions:

1. Preheat the oven to 400°F
2. Pour the olive oil into a large baking dish.
3. In the baking dish, combine the rosemary, oregano, garlic, red pepper flakes, salt, black pepper, and half of the sliced lemons.
4. Bake until fragrant (about 10 minutes). Meanwhile, wash and chop the broccoli into bite-size florets.
5. Remove the baking dish from the oven — Layer the broccoli and shrimp over the top of the herb mix. Gently toss until everything coats evenly.
6. Top with the remaining lemon slices and bake until the shrimp are pink and opaque.
7. Meanwhile, bring a large pot of water to a boil and cook the pasta according to the package directions for al dente (firm to the bite).
8. Add the cooked pasta to the baking dish after removing it from the oven.
9. Gently toss to combine thoroughly.
10. Serve immediately.

Nutrition Facts Per Serving

Calories 460, Total Fat 20g, Saturated Fat 3g, Total Carbs 51g, Protein 20g, Fiber:4g, Sodium: 520mg

Baked Oysters with Vegetables

Prep time: 30 minutes, Cook time: 15 to 17 minutes, Serves 2

Ingredients:

- 2 cups coarse salt, for holding the oysters
- 1 dozen fresh oysters, scrubbed
- 1 tablespoon almond butter
- ¼ cup finely chopped scallions, both white and green parts
- ½ cup finely chopped artichoke hearts

- ¼ cup finely chopped red bell pepper
- 1 garlic clove, minced
- 1 tablespoon finely chopped fresh parsley
- Zest and juice of ½ lemon
- Pinch salt
- Freshly ground black pepper, to taste

Instructions:
1. Pour the salt into a baking dish and spread to evenly fill the bottom of the dish.
2. Prepare a clean work surface to shuck the oysters. Using a shucking knife, insert the blade at the joint of the shell, where it hinges open and shut. Firmly apply pressure to pop the blade in, and work the knife around the shell to open. Discard the empty half of the shell. Using the knife, gently loosen the oyster, and remove any shell particles. Set the oysters in their shells on the salt, being careful not to spill the juices.
3. Preheat the oven to 425ºF (220ºC).
4. Heat the almond butter in a large skillet over medium heat. Add the scallions, artichoke hearts, and bell pepper, and cook for 5 to 7 minutes. Add the garlic and cook for 1 minute more.
5. Remove from the heat and stir in the parsley, lemon zest and juice, and season to taste with salt and pepper.
6. Divide the vegetable mixture evenly among the oysters. Bake in the preheated oven for 10 to 12 minutes, or until the vegetables are lightly browned. Serve warm.

Nutrition Facts Per Serving
calories: 135, fat: 7.2g, protein: 6.0g, carbs: 10.7g, fiber: 2.0g, sodium: 280mg

Pickled Herring

Prep time: 10 minutes, cook time: 30 minutes; Serves 4

Ingredients:
- 4 whole herring fillets, scaled, filleted, and trimmed
- 2 cups of water
- ½ sweet onion, thinly sliced
- ½ cup white vinegar
- 2 thyme sprigs
- 1 tablespoon granulated sugar
- 1 teaspoon of sea salt
- ¼ teaspoon black peppercorns

Instructions:
1. Preheat the oven to 350°F
2. Place the herring fillets in a 9-by-13-inch baking dish.
3. Add the water, onion, white vinegar, thyme, sugar, salt, and peppercorns.
4. Cover the baking dish with foil and bake the fish until tender, 25 to 30 minutes.
5. Cool before serving.

Nutrition Facts Per Serving
Calories 277, Total Fat 15g, Saturated Fat 4g, Total Carbs 5g, Protein 29g, Fiber:0g, Sodium:482mg

CHAPTER
5

Vegetarian Mains Recipes

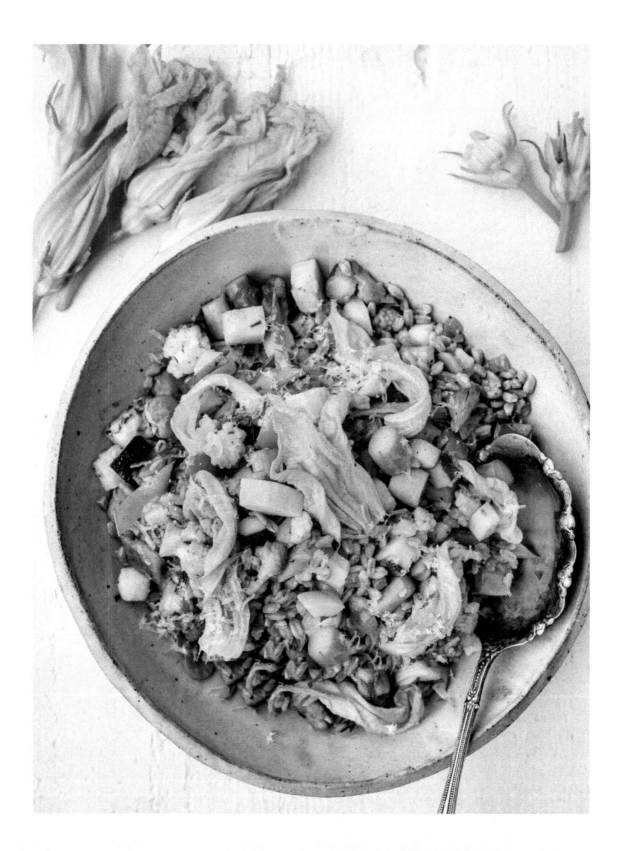

Succotash

Prep time: 10 minutes, cook time: 20 minutes; Serves 4

Ingredients:

- 2 tablespoons olive oil
- 1 sweet onion, finely chopped
- 1 tablespoon minced garlic
- 2 (15-ounce) cans diced sodium-free tomatoes, undrained
- 2 cups shelled edamame
- 2 cups corn
- 1 orange bell pepper, seeded and diced
- Sea salt and black pepper for seasoning
- 2 tablespoons finely chopped fresh parsley, for garnish

Instructions:

1. Heat the olive oil in a skillet over medium-high heat.
2. Sauté the onion and garlic until softened, about 3 minutes.
3. Add the tomatoes, edamame, corn, and bell pepper.
4. When it boils, reduce the heat and simmer until the vegetables are tender.
5. Season accordingly and serve topped with parsley.

Nutrition Facts Per Serving

Calories 265, Total Fat 12g, Saturated Fat 2g, Total Carbs 27g, Protein 11g, Fiber:6g, Sodium:101 mg

Cauliflower Steaks

Prep time: 10 minutes, cook time: 16 minutes; Serves 4

Ingredients:

- 1 large head cauliflower, sliced into 6 (1-inch-thick) steaks
- 2 tablespoons olive oil, divided
- ½ teaspoon smoked paprika
- ½ teaspoon kosher salt
- ¼ teaspoon cayenne pepper
- Balsamic Roasted Tomatoes

Instructions:

1. Rub both sides of the cauliflower steaks lightly with one tablespoon of olive oil, and sprinkle on both sides with the paprika, salt, and cayenne.
2. Heat the remaining one tablespoon of olive oil in a large sauté pan over medium-high heat. Arrange the cauliflower steaks in the pan, including any extra florets. You may need to cook the steaks in two batches.
3. Cook the cauliflower until slightly crisped, about 3 minutes per side. Reduce the heat to medium and continue to cook until the cauliflower is tender when pierced with a sharp knife.
4. Serve the cauliflower steaks topped with the roasted tomatoes.

Nutrition Facts Per Serving

Calories 114, Total Fat 8g, Total Carbs11g, Protein 4g, Sugar: 5g, Fiber: 5g, Sodium: 354mg

Whole- Wheat Flatbreads

Prep time: 15 minutes, cook time: 15 minutes; Serves 4

Ingredients:

- ⅔ cup of warm water
- 1 teaspoon salt
- ¼ cup olive oil
- 2 cups white whole-wheat flour
- Pinch dried herbs (rosemary, basil, oregano, or others; optional)

Instructions:

1. In a large bowl, stir together the warm water and salt until the salt dissolves. Stir in the olive oil.
2. Add the flour and work it with your hands until the moisture distributes, and the dough comes together. Knead the dough in the bowl for 3 to 4 minutes. Let it rest for 15 minutes.
3. Cut the dough into four pieces. Place each portion between two sheets of parchment paper and use a rolling pin to roll it as thin as possible. It'll puff up while cooking, so try to roll it into a super-thin sheet.
4. Sprinkle with the herbs, if using.
5. Heat a large nonstick skillet over medium heat and cook each piece for 2 to 3 minutes per side. You won't need any oil—as long as you use a nonstick pan, you shouldn't have any trouble flipping the flatbreads. Be sure not to overcook, or they'll get crispy.
6. Let cool and store in an airtight container until you're ready to use them.

Nutrition Facts Per Serving

Calories 158, Total Fat 13g, Total Carbs 11g, Protein 2g, Sugar:1g, Fiber:2g, Sodium:581mg

Roasted Chickpeas

Prep time: 10 minutes, cook time: 30 minutes; Serves 4

Ingredients:

- 2 (15-ounce) cans chickpeas, drained and rinsed
- 1 tablespoon olive oil
- ½ teaspoon salt
- Garlic powder, cumin, chili powder, or any spices you like

Instructions:

1. Preheat the oven to 450°F
2. In a large bowl, toss the chickpeas and olive oil together until the chickpeas are well coated.
3. Sprinkle with the salt and any other spices you'd like to use.
4. Line a baking sheet with parchment paper and spread the chickpeas out in a single layer.
5. Bake for fifteen minutes, then stir the chickpeas and continue to bake for 10 minutes more until the chickpeas become brown and crispy.

Nutrition Facts Per Serving

Calories 316, Total Fat 6g, Saturated Fat, Total Carbs 54g, Protein 12g, Sugar:0g, Fiber:11g, Sodium:1008mg

Mexican Salsa

Prep time: 5 minutes, chill time: 1 hour; serves 6

Ingredients:
- 4 firm tomatoes (large)
- 1 fresh jalapeno
- 2 tablespoons fresh cilantro (chopped)
- ½ red onion (medium, diced)
- 1 lime
- Salt and black pepper to taste

Instructions:
1. Skin and seed the tomatoes.
2. Halve the jalapeno and remove the stem and seeds.
3. Cut the tomatoes and jalapeno into small pieces.
4. Add the cut veggies to a medium-size bowl.
5. Chop the cilantro and red onion into tiny bits and add to the bowl.
6. Juice the lime into the bowl and stir the ingredients well.
7. Season the mixture to taste with salt and black pepper.
8. After all the ingredients are combined, let it sit in the fridge for one hour before serving.
9. Enjoy!

Nutrition Facts Per Serving
Calories 30, Total Fat, Total Carbs 6.1g, Protein 0.8g, Sugar: 4g, Fiber: 2.1g,)

Zucchini Noodles

Prep time: 10 minutes, cook time: 10 minutes; Serves 4

Ingredients:
- 4 medium zucchini
- Salt to taste
- 1 teaspoon olive oil

Instructions:
1. Slice the ends of the zucchini, so you have a flat surface on each end.
2. Spiralize into strands, cutting them every 6 inches.
3. Discard the "seedy" strands from the center of the zucchini to avoid making the rest of your strands soggy.
4. Sprinkle the noodles with a pinch of salt and let them sit in a colander for at least 10 minutes to help get rid of some of the excess moisture.
5. In a large nonstick skillet over medium heat, sauté the zucchini with the olive oil for 2 to 3 minutes. Be careful not to overcook, or the noodles will get soggy.
6. Drain any excess moisture from the bottom of the skillet.
7. Add your favorite sauce or seasoning and toss it with the noodles. Serve immediately.

Nutrition Facts Per Serving
Calories 41, Total Fat 2g, Total Carbs 7g, Protein 2g, Sugar:3g, Fiber:2g, Sodium:58mg

Cauliflower Rice

Prep time: 10 minutes, cook time: 10 minutes; Serves 4

Ingredients:

- 1 large head cauliflower
- 1 tablespoon olive oil

Instructions:

1. Tear off any green leaves that are still on the cauliflower then, using a sharp knife; chop the head into four large pieces.
2. In a large bowl using a box grater, grate the cauliflower into rice-size bits. Or you can finely chop it in a food processor.
3. Heat the olive oil in a large nonstick skillet over medium heat. Add the cauliflower and cook for 6 minutes, frequently stirring, until it starts to soften.
4. Drain any excess moisture from the skillet.
5. Add any seasoning you like and serve immediately.

Nutrition Facts Per Serving

Calories 83, Total Fat 4g, Saturated Fat, Total Carbs 11g, Protein 4g, Sugar:5g, Fiber:5g, Sodium:63mg

Quinoa–Sweet Potato Stew

Prep time: 10 minutes, cook time: 30 minutes; Serves 4

Ingredients:

- 1 tablespoon olive oil
- 1 sweet onion, finely chopped
- 1 tablespoon minced garlic
- 1 (15-ounce) can diced tomatoes, undrained
- 1 (15-ounce) can lentils, drained and rinsed
- 2 large sweet potatoes, peeled and diced
- ½ cup of water
- 2 cups green beans cut into 2-inch pieces
- 2 cups cooked quinoa
- Sea salt, for seasoning
- Freshly ground black pepper, for seasoning

Instructions:

1. In a large saucepan, heat the olive oil over medium-high heat.
2. Sauté the onion and garlic until softened, about 3 minutes.
3. Add the tomatoes, lentils, sweet potatoes, and water.
4. Bring the liquid to a boil and then reduce the heat to low, simmering until the sweet potatoes are tender about 20 minutes.
5. Stir in the green beans and quinoa and cook 5 minutes to heat through.
6. Season accordingly and serve immediately

Nutrition Facts Per Serving

Calories 362, Total Fat 6g, Saturated Fat 1g, Total Carbs, Protein 16g, Fiber:16g, Sodium:94mg

Chickpea-Stuffed Sweet Potatoes

Prep time: 10 minutes, cook time: 40 minutes; Serves 4

Ingredients:

- 4 large sweet potatoes
- 1 (14.5-ounce) can chickpeas, drained and rinsed
- ½ teaspoon ground cumin
- ½ teaspoon red pepper flakes
- ½ teaspoon smoked paprika
- ¼ teaspoon dried sage
- Salt and freshly ground black pepper
- 1 tablespoon extra-virgin olive oil
- ½ bunch curly parsley, large stems removed
- 1 cup halved cherry tomatoes
- ½ red onion, finely diced
- 2 garlic cloves, minced
- Juice of 1 lemon
- 1 cup prepared hummus
- ½ cup sunflower seeds, roasted and salted

Instructions:

1. Preheat the oven to 400°F
2. Wash the sweet potatoes thoroughly and pierce with a knife. Put on a baking sheet and bake for 40 minutes or until tender.
3. Dry the chickpeas and add to a small bowl with the cumin, red pepper flakes, smoked paprika, and sage. Season with salt and pepper, and then add the olive oil and mix.
4. Spread on a baking sheet and place it in the oven when 30 minutes are remaining on the potatoes.
5. Meanwhile, make a tomato-parsley salad: Coarsely chop the parsley. Add to the same small bowl along with the cherry tomatoes, onion, garlic, and lemon juice. Stir to combine, and then chill until ready to serve. When the sweet potatoes and chickpeas are finished baking, remove from the oven and allow cooling for about 10 minutes.
6. Cut each potato into two, then fluff with a fork.
7. To serve, spoon ¼ cup of hummus per potato, distributing evenly on each half. Then add the tomato-parsley salad, chickpeas, and sunflower seeds.
8. Serve immediately.

Nutrition Facts Per Serving

Calories 430, Total Fat 15g, Saturated Fat 2g, Total Carbs 63g, Protein 15g, Sugar:13g, Fiber:15g, Sodium:490mg

Quinoa Stuffed Sweet Potato

Prep time: 10 minutes, cook time: 1 hour; serves 4

Ingredients:

- 4 sweet potatoes
- Kosher salt
- Freshly ground black pepper
- ¾ cup quinoa, rinsed
- ½ cup crumbled goat cheese
- 2 tablespoons honey
- 2 tablespoons chopped fresh rosemary

Instructions:

1. Preheat the oven to 400°F. Line a baking sheet with aluminum foil or parchment paper.
2. Pierce the sweet potatoes a few times with a fork.
3. Season with salt and black pepper and transfer to the prepared baking sheet and bake for 40 minutes, or until sweet potatoes are slightly soft. While the sweet potatoes are in the oven, cook the quinoa according to the package instructions.
4. In a medium mixing bowl, combine the goat cheese, honey, and rosemary, and season with salt and black pepper.
5. Once the quinoa is well cooked, fold it into the goat cheese mixture.
6. Remove the sweet potatoes from the oven, but leave it on. When the sweet potatoes are cold enough, carefully cut each open lengthwise.
7. Scoop out each sweet potato and stuff it with the quinoa and goat cheese mixture.
8. Place back in the oven at 400°F for another 10 to 15 minutes, or until the cheese is gooey, golden, and slightly melted.

Nutrition Facts Per Serving

Calories 331, Total Fat 7g, Saturated Fat 4g, Total Carbs 57g, Protein 11g, Sugar:14g, Fiber:6g, Sodium:162mg

CHAPTER 6

Soups and Salads Recipes

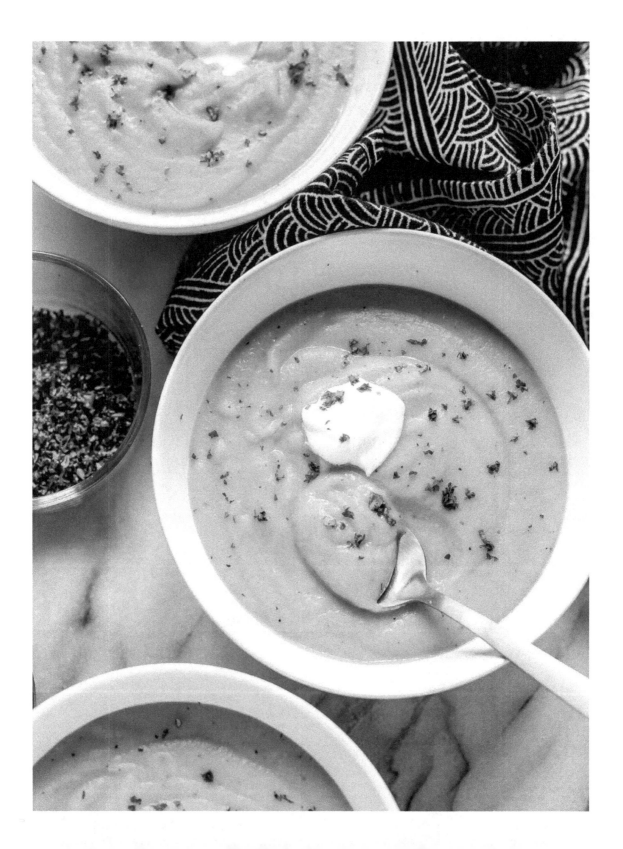

Cantaloupe Cold soup

Prep time: 10 minutes, Chill time: 1 Hour; Serves 4

Ingredients:

- 2 cantaloupes, seeded, peeled, and diced
- 1 cucumber, diced
- 1 tablespoon apple cider vinegar
- 1 teaspoon of grated fresh ginger
- 2 shallots, finely chopped
- 2 tablespoons finely chopped fresh mint

Instructions:

1. In a food processor, purée the cantaloupes, cucumber, vinegar, ginger, and shallots until smooth.
2. Transfer the soup to a container and chill in the refrigerator, about an hour.
3. Serve topped with fresh mint.

Nutrition Facts Per Serving

Calories 155, Total Fat 1g, Saturated Fat 0g, Total Carbs37g, Protein4g, Fiber:4g, Sodium:68mg

Potato and Salmon Soup

Prep time: 10 minutes, cook time: 30 minutes; Serves 4

Ingredients:

- 1 tablespoon olive oil
- 3 leeks, trimmed, washed, and roughly chopped
- ½ sweet onion, roughly chopped
- 6 cups low-sodium vegetable stock
- 4 large russet potatoes, peeled and
- diced
- ¼ cup coconut cream
- 8 ounces smoked salmon, roughly chopped
- Sea salt and black pepper for seasoning

Instructions:

1. In a large saucepan, heat the olive oil over medium-high heat.
2. Sauté the leeks and onion until soft and translucent, for about five minutes
3. Stir in the vegetable stock and potatoes and bring to a boil.
4. Reduce the heat, cover, and simmer until the potatoes are tender about 20 minutes.
5. In a food processor, purée the soup until smooth, then return it to the saucepan, and whisk in the coconut cream and smoked salmon.
6. Season with salt and pepper and serve.

Nutrition Facts Per Serving

Calories 409, Total Fat 16g, Saturated Fat 9g, Total Carbs 50g, Protein 16g, Fiber:7g, Sodium:1528mg

Shrimp Ginger Soup

Prep time: 10 minutes, cook time: 20 minutes; Serves 4

Ingredients:

- 1 tablespoon olive oil
- 2 teaspoons minced garlic
- 2 teaspoons grated fresh ginger
- 3 cups low-sodium vegetable stock
- 1 cup full-fat coconut milk
- 2 cups shredded kale
- 1 pound shrimp, peeled, deveined, and chopped into ¼-inch pieces
- Sea salt and black pepper for seasoning

Instructions:

1. Over medium heat, heat the olive oil in a saucepan.
2. Sauté the garlic and ginger until softened, about 2 minutes.
3. Add the vegetable stock and coconut milk.
4. Boil the soup then add the kale and shrimp.
5. Simmer the soup until the shrimp cook through (about 5 minutes).
6. Season accordingly, and then serve.

Nutrition Facts Per Serving

Calories309, Total Fat 19g, Saturated Fat14g, Total Carbs 9g, Protein, Sugar:26g, Fiber:2g, Sodium:437 mg

Carrot Soup

Prep time: 8 minutes, cook time: 45 minutes; Serves 4

Ingredients:

- 1 tablespoon olive oil
- 1 sweet onion, finely chopped
- 2 teaspoons minced garlic
- 6 carrots, peeled and finely chopped
- 1 sweet potato, peeled and diced
- 6 cups low-sodium vegetable stock
- ½ teaspoon ground nutmeg
- ½ cup coconut cream
- Sea salt, and freshly ground black for seasoning

Instructions:

1. In a large saucepan, heat the olive oil over medium heat.
2. Add the onion and garlic and sauté until softened, about 3 minutes.
3. Add the carrots, sweet potato, vegetable stock, and nutmeg.
4. Bring the soup to a boil and then reduce the heat to low and simmer the soup until the vegetables are soft, about 30 minutes.
5. In a food processor, purée the soup in batches until smooth
6. Return the puréed soup to the pot and stir in the coconut cream.
7. Season with salt and pepper and serve.

Nutrition Facts Per Serving

Calories333, Total Fat 22g, Saturated Fat16g, Total Carbs 28g, Protein 4g, Fiber:4g, Sodium: 484mg

Whitefish Soup

Prep time: 10 minutes, cook time: 15 minutes; Serves 4

Ingredients:
- 6 cups low-sodium vegetable stock
- 2 tablespoons white miso paste
- 1 tablespoon grated fresh ginger
- 1 pound whitefish, thinly sliced
- 2 cups roughly chopped Swiss chard, thoroughly washed

Instructions:
1. In a saucepan, boil the vegetable stock over medium-high heat.
2. Stir in the miso paste and ginger and simmer for 5 minutes.
3. Add the whitefish and simmer until just cooked through about 5 minutes.
4. Stir in the chard and simmer until wilted, about 3 minutes.
5. Serve immediately.

Nutrition Facts Per Serving

Calories 226, Total Fat 8g, Saturated Fat 1g, Total Carbs 4g, Protein 29g, Fiber:0g, Sodium:1362mg

Cobb Salad

Prep time: 10 minutes, cook time: 10 minutes; Serves 4

Ingredients:
- 6 cups roughly chopped romaine
- 4 hard-boiled eggs, diced
- 3 tomatoes, diced
- 1 medium ripe avocado, pitted and diced
- ¼ cup store-bought Asian-style dressing
- For the dressing
- ¼ cup olive oil,
- 3 tablespoons sesame oil
- ⅓ Cup of rice vinegar
- 2 tablespoons soy sauce
- 2 tablespoons honey
- 1 teaspoon minced garlic

Instructions:
1. Spread the romaine on a platter or 4 plates.
2. Arrange the eggs, tomato, and avocado on the romaine in rows to create an appealing pattern.
3. Drizzle with the dressing and serve.
4. For the dressing
5. Whisk together olive oil, sesame oil, rice vinegar soy sauce, honey, and minced garlic.

Nutrition Facts Per Serving

Calories293, Total Fat 21g, Saturated Fat 4g, Total Carbs 14g, Protein 7g, Fiber:4g, Sodium: 356mg

Tomato and Crab Salad

Prep time: 10 minutes; Serves 4

Ingredients:
- 1 fennel bulb, shredded
- 3 large tomatoes, diced
- 1 cucumber, halved lengthwise and thinly sliced
- 12 ounces crabmeat
- ½ cup store-bought creamy ranch dressing

Instructions:
1. In a mixing bowl, combine the fennel, tomatoes, and cucumber.
2. Arrange the salad on four plates and divide the crab meat evenly between them.
3. Drizzle the salad with dressing and serve.

Nutrition Facts Per Serving
Calories 271, Total Fat 17g, Saturated Fat 1g, Total Carbs 16g, Protein 14g, Fiber: 4g, Sodium:593mg

Avocado and Quinoa Salad

Prep time: 10 minutes, cook time: 10 minutes; Serves 4

Ingredients:
- 2 navel oranges
- ¼ cup olive oil
- ¼ teaspoon salt
- A Pinch of freshly ground black pepper
- 8 cups spinach
- 2 avocados, diced
- ¼ cup sliced almonds
- 1 cup cooked quinoa, cooled

Instructions:
1. Segment the oranges: Slice off the top, bottom, and peel of each.
2. Over a medium bowl, cut into each orange between the membranes to remove the segments of flesh. Set aside the orange segments.
3. Squeeze what remains of the oranges to release the rest of their juice into the bowl.
4. Combine the olive oil with the orange juice, and add the salt and pepper. Set aside.
5. Put the spinach in a large bowl then add the avocados. Top with the orange segments, almonds, and quinoa.
6. Toss with the dressing just before serving.

Nutrition Facts Per Serving
Calories 409, Total Fat 31g, Total Carbs 32g, Protein 8g, Sugar:7g, Fiber:11g, Sodium: 203mg

Basil Guacamole

Prep time: 10 minutes; Serves 3

Ingredients:
- 1 large avocado, pitted
- 2 cups frozen chopped spinach, thawed and liquid squeezed out
- 1 tomato, finely chopped
- 1 tablespoon finely chopped fresh basil
- Juice and zest of ½ a lemon
- Sea salt and black pepper for seasoning

Instructions:
1. In a medium bowl, mash the avocado with a potato masher or fork until chunky.
2. Stir in the spinach, tomato, basil, lemon juice, and lemon zest until well combined.
3. Season with salt and pepper
4. Serve immediately or refrigerate in a resealable container for up to 3 days.

Nutrition Facts Per Serving

Calories54, Total Fat 5g, Saturated Fat 1g, Total Carbs 3g, Protein 1g, Fiber:2g, Sodium51mg

Tomato and Chickpea Salad

Prep time: 10 minutes, cook time: 10 minutes; Serves 4

Ingredients:
- 1 pound tomatoes
- 2 medium cucumbers
- 2 (15-ounce) cans chickpeas, drained and rinsed
- ¼ cup crumbled feta cheese
- ¼ cup chopped fresh dill
- 2 tablespoons olive oil
- 2 teaspoons balsamic vinegar
- Salt and black pepper to taste

Instructions:
1. Cut the tomatoes into large chunks.
2. Slice the cucumber into small quarters.
3. Combine the tomatoes, cucumbers, and chickpeas in a large bowl.
4. Sprinkle with the feta and dill.
5. Drizzle with olive oil and vinegar and season accordingly.

Nutrition Facts Per Serving

Calories 421, Total Fat 12g, Total Carbs 66g, Protein 16g, Sugar:6g, Fiber:13g, Sodium:876mg

CHAPTER 7

Snacks and Sides Recipes

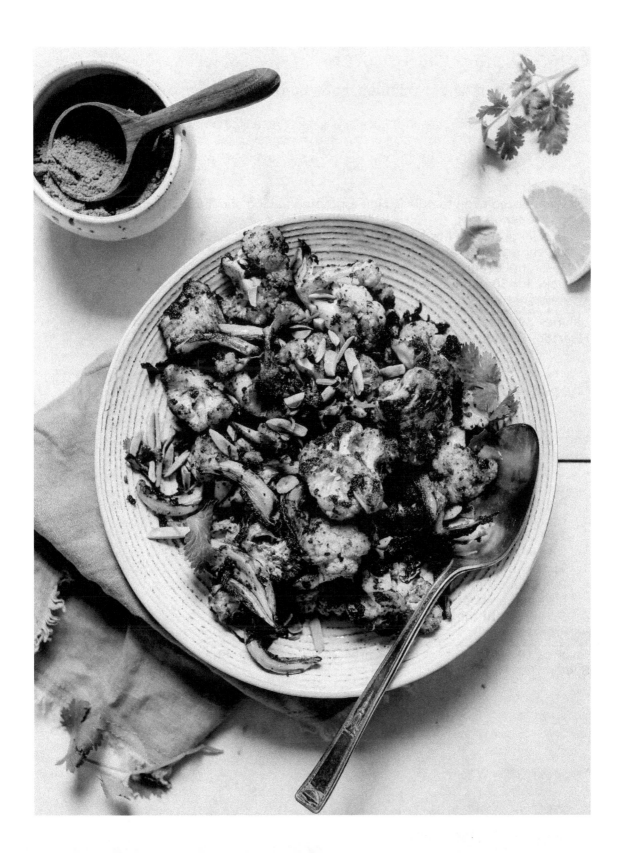

Crispy Baked Cauliflower

Prep time: 5 minutes, cook time: 30 minutes; Serves 4

Ingredients:

- 1 head cauliflower, cut into florets
- 1 tablespoon olive oil
- 2 teaspoons ground turmeric
- 1 teaspoon ground cumin
- ½ teaspoon ground cayenne pepper
- Kosher salt
- Freshly ground black pepper

Instructions:

1. Preheat the oven to 400°F. Line a rimmed baking sheet with aluminum foil or parchment paper.
2. In a large mixing bowl, combine the cauliflower florets, olive oil, turmeric, cumin, cayenne pepper, and salt and black pepper to taste.
3. Toss until evenly coated and transfer to the prepared baking sheet.
4. Bake for 30 minutes, until the cauliflower browns and slightly crispy.

Nutrition Facts Per Serving

Calories 89, Total Fat 4g, Saturated Fat 1g, Total Carbs 12g, Protein 4g, Sugar:5g, Fiber:6g, Sodium:103mg

Sweet Potato Fries

Prep time: 10 minutes, cook time: 20 minutes; Serves 4

Ingredients:

- 2 large sweet potatoes
- 1 tablespoon olive oil
- 4 garlic cloves, minced
- 1 teaspoon salt

Instructions:

1. Preheat the oven to 450°F then spray a nonstick baking sheet with nonstick cooking spray.
2. Peel the potatoes and cut them into wedges.
3. In a large bowl, toss the potato wedges with the olive oil.
4. Spread them evenly on the prepared baking sheet.
5. Roast for 10 minutes, flip, and continue to roast for 10 minutes more or until browned on both sides.
6. Sprinkle with the garlic and salt before serving.

Nutrition Facts Per Serving

Calories 101, Total Fat 4g, Total Carbs 12g, Protein 1g, Sugar:4g, Fiber:2g, Sodium:604mg

Tuna Stuffed Peppers

Prep time: 10 minutes; Serves 4

Ingredients:
- 1 (5-ounce) can of tuna, drained
- ¼ cup hummus
- 1 celery stalk, finely chopped
- ¼ red onion, finely chopped
- 12 tricolored mini bell peppers, seeded, deveined, and halved plus
- 1 mini bell pepper, seeded, deveined, and finely chopped

Instructions:
1. In a mixing bowl, combine the tuna, hummus, celery, and red onion.
2. Place the pepper halves on a serving tray.
3. Using a spoon, stuff the mini pepper halves with the tuna-hummus mixture.
4. Sprinkle with the chopped mini pepper.

Nutrition Facts Per Serving

Calories 193, Total Fat 2g, Saturated Fat 0g, Total Carbs 18g, Protein 24g, Sugar 9g, Fiber: 4g, Sodium:380mg

Salmon Pâté

Prep time: 20 minutes; Serves 6

Ingredients:
- 1 cup low-fat cream cheese
- ½ cup ricotta cheese
- Juice and zest of 1 lime
- 1 tablespoon chopped fresh dill
- 6 ounces smoked salmon

Instructions:
1. In a food processor, pulse the cream cheese and ricotta until smooth.
2. Add the lime juice, lime zest, and dill, and pulse until blended.
3. Add the salmon and pulse until combined but still chunky.
4. Transfer the pâté to a container and store it in the refrigerator for up to 1 week.

Nutrition Facts Per Serving

Calories 178, Total Fat 6g, Saturated Fat 4g, Total Carbs 8g, Protein 19g, Fiber:0g, Sodium:831mg

Apple Snack

Prep time: 6 minutes; Serves 1

Ingredients:
- 1 Granny Smith apple
- 1½ tablespoons peanut butter
- ½ tablespoon hemp hearts
- 1 tablespoon mini chocolate chips
- 2 tablespoons dried cranberries

Instructions:
1. Lay the apple on its side and slice into ½-inch-thick rounds and remove the core from the center.

2. Use a butter knife to spread peanut butter onto each slice.
3. Top with the hemp hearts, chocolate chips, and cranberries, distributing evenly over each slice.
4. Serve immediately.

Nutrition Facts Per Serving
Calories 339, Total Fat 17g, Saturated Fat 4g, Total Carbs 45g, Protein 9g, Sugar 10g, Fiber:8g, Sodium:110mg

Roasted Brussels sprouts

Prep time: 5 minutes, cook time: 40 minutes; Serves 4

Ingredients:
- 3 cups Brussels sprouts, halved
- 1 apple, cored and diced
- ⅓ cup of unsweetened applesauce
- 2 tablespoons olive oil
- 1 tablespoon honey
- Kosher salt
- Freshly ground black pepper

Instructions:
1. Preheat the oven to 400°F then line a rimmed baking sheet with aluminum foil or parchment paper.
2. In a bowl, combine the Brussels sprouts, apple, applesauce, olive oil, and honey.
3. Season accordingly, and then transfer to the prepared baking sheet.
4. Bake until the Brussels sprouts brown slightly and crispy.

Nutrition Facts Per Serving
Calories 142, Total Fat 7g, Saturated Fat 1g, Total Carbs 20g, Protein 3g, Sugar:14g, Fiber:4g, Sodium:56mg

Roasted Broccoli

Prep time: 10 minutes, cook time: 10 minutes; Serves 4

Ingredients:
- 1 head broccoli
- 1 tablespoon olive oil
- Juice of 1 lemon
- ¼ teaspoon salt
- Pinch freshly ground black pepper
- ¼ cup slivered almonds

Instructions:
1. Preheat the oven to 425°F
2. Cut the broccoli florets into 1-inch pieces, discarding the woody stem.
3. In a large bowl, toss the broccoli with the olive oil, lemon juice, salt, and pepper.
4. Spread the broccoli pieces on a nonstick baking sheet and roast for 8 minutes, then flip the pieces over and sprinkle with the almonds.
5. Roast the broccoli and almonds together for 3 minutes more, until browned.

Nutrition Facts Per Serving
Calories 106, Total Fat 7g, Total Carbs 9g, Protein 5g, Sugar:2g, Fiber:4g, Sodium:187mg

Potted Salmon

Prep time: 10 minutes, Chill time: 2 Hours; Serves 4

Ingredients:
- ½ pound cooked salmon
- ½ cup plain low-fat Greek yogurt
- ¼ cup butter, melted
- Juice and zest from ½ a lemon
- 1 tablespoon finely chopped fresh dill
- Sea salt and black pepper for seasoning

Instructions:
1. In a medium bowl, mix the salmon, yogurt, butter, lemon juice, lemon zest, and dill until well combined.
2. Season with salt and pepper.
3. Chill the potted salmon for at least 2 hours before serving.
4. Store the potted salmon in a sealed container in the refrigerator for up to 1 week.

Nutrition Facts Per Serving

Calories 228, Total Fat 17g, Saturated Fat 8g, Total Carbs 2g, Protein 18g, Fiber:0g, Sodium:129mg

Fresh Pea Hummus

Prep time: 10 minutes, cook time: 7 minutes; Serves 2

Ingredients:
- 1 cup fresh shelled peas
- Coarse salt
- ¼ cup fresh cilantro (leaves and stems)
- 2 tablespoons tahini
- 2 tablespoons fresh lemon juice
- 1 small garlic clove, minced
- 1 teaspoon ground cumin
- Whole-grain crackers, for serving

Instructions:
1. Cook peas in a pot of salted water until tender. Drain; run under cold water to stop the cooking.
2. Pulse peas, cilantro, tahini, lemon juice, garlic, and cumin in the food processor until smooth.
3. Season with salt and serve with crackers.

Nutrition Facts Per Serving

Calories 74, Total Fat 4g, Saturated Fat 1g, Total Carbs 7g, Protein 3g, Fiber:2g

Spicy Edamame

Prep time: 5 minutes, cook time: 10 minutes; Serves 4

Ingredients:
- 1 pound frozen edamame still in pods
- 1 tablespoon olive oil
- 4 garlic cloves, pressed or minced
- ¼ teaspoon red pepper flakes
- Sea salt
- Soy sauce, for serving

Instructions:
1. Bring a pot of salted water to a boil, then add the edamame and boil until bright green and tender.
2. Heat the olive oil in a skillet over medium heat, then add the garlic and red pepper flakes, and cook for about six minutes.
3. Drain the edamame and add it to the skillet.
4. Stir to coat the edamame with the flavored oil.
5. Transfer to a serving bowl and season with sea salt.
6. Serve with soy sauce on the side for dipping.

Nutrition Facts Per Serving

Calories 211, Total Fat 11g, Total Carbs 16g, Protein 15g, Sugar 0g, Fiber:5g, Sodium:77mg

Edamame Hummus

Prep time: 10 minutes; Serves 4

Ingredients:
- 1 avocado
- 1½ cups frozen shelled edamame, thawed
- ¼ cup chopped fresh cilantro
- 1 scallion, cut into short pieces
- 1 teaspoon onion powder
- 2 tablespoons extra-virgin olive oil
- 1 tablespoon tahini
- Pinch salt
- Pinch freshly ground black pepper

Instructions:
1. Combine all of the listed ingredients in your food processor.
2. Pulse until the mixture becomes smooth.

Nutrition Facts Per Serving

Calories 211, Total Fat 17g, Saturated Fat 25g, Total Carbs 10g, Protein 8g, Sugar: 2g, Fiber: 6g, Sodium:50mg

CHAPTER 8

Pasta, Rice and Grains Recipes

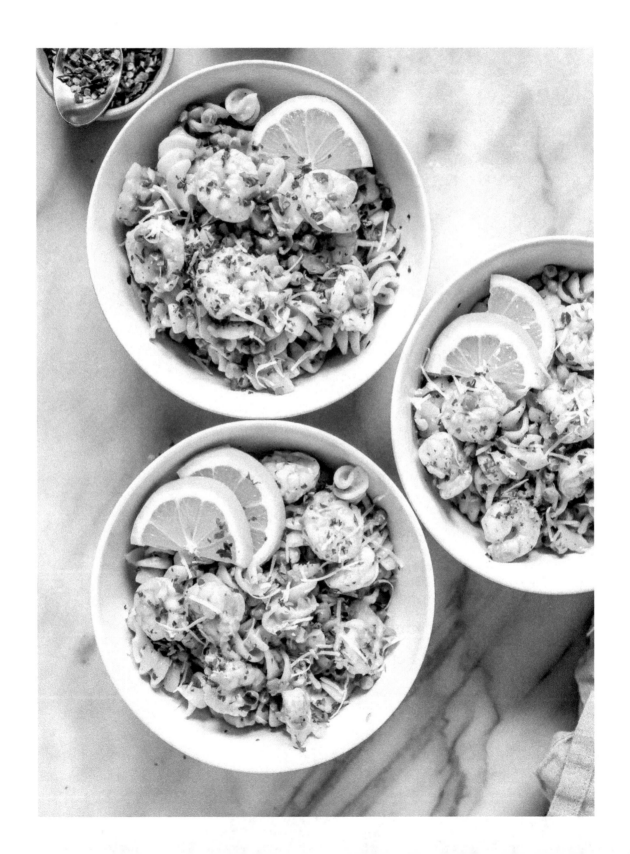

Spaghetti with Radicchio

Prep time: 10 minutes, cook time: 20 minutes; Serves 4

Ingredients:

- 8-ounces dry spaghetti
- 2 tablespoons olive oil
- 1 tablespoon minced garlic
- 2 radicchio heads, shredded
- ¼ cup balsamic vinegar
- Pinch red pepper flakes
- Sea salt, for seasoning
- 2 tablespoons finely chopped fresh parsley

Instructions:

1. Cook the pasta according to the package instructions.
2. While the pasta is cooking, heat the olive oil in a large skillet over medium-high heat.
3. Sauté the garlic until softened, about 2 minutes.
4. Add the shredded radicchio and sauté until tender, 5 minutes.
5. Stir in the balsamic vinegar and red pepper flakes and sauté 3 to 4 minutes more.
6. Add the cooked pasta and combine well.
7. Season with salt and serve topped with parsley.

`Nutrition Facts Per Serving`

Calories 275, Total Fat 8g, Saturated Fat 1g, Total Carbs 45g, Protein 9g, Sugar: Fiber:1g, Sodium:74mg

Rice with Shrimp

Prep time: 10 minutes, cook time: 37 minutes; Serves 4

Ingredients:

- 1 tablespoon olive oil
- 1 tablespoon grated fresh ginger
- 1 teaspoon minced garlic
- 1 cup brown basmati rice
- 2 cups of water
- 2 cups roughly chopped peeled, cooked shrimp
- 1 cup frozen sweet peas, thawed
- Juice and zest of 1 lime
- Sea salt, for seasoning
- Freshly ground black pepper, for seasoning

Instructions:

1. Heat the olive oil in a pan over medium heat.
2. Sauté the ginger and garlic until softened (about two minutes).
3. Add the rice and sauté for three minutes.
4. Stir in the water, and then reduce the heat to low so that the rice simmers. Simmer until the rice is tender.
5. Stir in the shrimp, peas, lime juice, and lime zest. Let stand 5 minutes, covered.
6. Season with salt and pepper and serve.

`Nutrition Facts Per Serving`

Calories 213, Total Fat 5g, Saturated Fat 1g, Total Carbs 22g, Protein 21g, Fiber:2g, Sodium:447mg

Pecan Wild Rice

Prep time: 10 minutes, cook time: 45 minutes; Serves 4

Ingredients:

- 2 tablespoons olive oil
- 2 cups sliced wild mushrooms
- ½ sweet onion, finely chopped
- 2 teaspoons minced garlic
- 1 cup uncooked brown basmati wild rice mixture
- 2 cups low-sodium vegetable stock
- Sea salt, for seasoning
- Freshly ground black pepper, for seasoning
- ½ cup chopped pecans
- 1 teaspoon finely chopped fresh thyme

Instructions:

1. Heat the olive oil in a pan over medium heat.
2. Sauté the mushrooms, onion, and garlic until golden and soft, about 7 minutes
3. Add in the rice and vegetable stock and let it boil.
4. Reduce the heat and simmer, covered, until the liquid is absorbed and the rice is tender.
5. Season accordingly and serve topped with pecans and thyme.

Nutrition Facts Per Serving

Calories331, Total Fat 16g, Saturated Fat 3g, Total Carbs 41g, Protein 9g, Fiber:3g, Sodium:67mg

Rustic Pasta

Prep time: 10 minutes, cook time: 20 minutes; Serves 4

Ingredients:

- 2 tomatoes, sliced
- 3 tablespoon + 1 teaspoon extra virgin olive oil, divided
- 1 small clove garlic, finely grated
- ¼ cup fresh basil leaves, sliced
- Sea salt and black pepper to taste
- 1 cup chickpeas, cooked
- ¼ cup pine nuts, raw
- 2 tablespoons nutritional yeast
- ¼ teaspoon garlic powder
- ½ teaspoon lemon zest
- 1 lb pasta, cooked

Instructions:

1. Add tomatoes to a bowl. Add in 3 tablespoons of oil, garlic, basil, olive oil, basil, salt, and pepper. Cover the bowl and set it aside for 4 hours.
2. Preheat oven to 400 F. Add chickpeas to a baking dish and toss them with the remaining oil, salt, and pepper.
3. Bake for 12 minutes. Add in pine nuts and roast for another 6 minutes. Take out and let them cool.
4. Add roasted chickpeas and pine nuts to a food processor. Add in all remaining ingredients except pasta, tomatoes, and roasted chickpeas and pine nut puree.
5. Pulse until the mixture is crumbly. Add pasta, roasted chickpeas, and pine nut puree and tomatoes to a bowl.
6. Toss well and serve.

Nutrition Facts Per Serving

Calories 678, Total Fat 22.2g, Saturated Fat 2.6g, Total Carbs 97.5g, Protein 25.5g, Sugar:7.3g, Fiber:10.5g, Sodium:46mg, Potassium907mg

Spicy Noodles

Ingredients:

- 8 ounces whole-wheat spaghetti noodles
- 1½ tablespoons soy sauce
- 1½ tablespoons sesame oil
- 2 teaspoons rice vinegar
- 1½ tablespoons honey
- ¼ teaspoon sriracha, plus more to taste
- 2 cups shelled edamame

Instructions:

1. Bring a large pot of water to a boil. Cook the whole-wheat spaghetti noodles according to the package directions.
2. While the noodles cook, whisk together the soy sauce, sesame oil, vinegar, honey, and sriracha in a small bowl.
3. Drain the noodles, and then return them to the pot.
4. Stir in the sauce and edamame, and continue to cook over medium heat for 2 minutes, stirring until the sauce thickens and the edamame is warm.

Nutrition Facts Per Serving

Calories 352, Total Fat 9g, Total Carbs 56g, Protein 16g, Sugar: 8g, Fiber:2g, Sodium:801mg

Garlic Alfredo Pasta

Prep time: 10 minutes, cook time: 20 minutes; Serves 4

Ingredients:

- 16-ounce Brussels sprouts halved
- 2 tablespoon olive oil
- 1 pinch each sea salt and black pepper
- Sauce + pasta:
- 3 tablespoon olive oil
- 4 large cloves garlic, chopped
- 1/3 cup dry white wine
- 4 tablespoon cornstarch
- ¾ cup unsweetened almond milk
- 4 tablespoon yeast
- Sea salt and black pepper, to taste
- ¼ cup vegan parmesan cheese
- 10-ounce pasta, cooked

Instructions:

1. Preheat oven to 400 F.
2. Place Brussels sprouts on a baking sheet.
3. Drizzle with oil, salt, and pepper and toss. Spread the sprouts in a single layer and set aside. Now, to make the pasta sauce, add oil and garlic in a skillet over medium heat and sauté for 3 minutes.
4. Add in the wine and stir for 2 minutes. Add cornstarch, almond milk, yeast, salt, pepper, and cheese and whisk continuously.
5. Bake Brussels sprouts for 15 minutes and once done, add pasta to the skillet and mix them with the sauce.
6. Serve and enjoy.

Nutrition Facts Per Serving

Calories 509, Total Fat 18.5g, Saturated Fat 2.4g, Total Carbs 75.4g, Protein 12.4g, Sugar:2.9g, Fiber:7.7g, Sodium:450mg, Potassium410mg

Brown Rice Stir Fry

Prep time: 10 minutes, cook time: 30 minutes; Serves 4

Ingredients:
- ½ cup brown rice, cooked
- 1 cup red cabbage, chopped
- 1 cup broccoli, chopped
- ½ red bell pepper, chopped
- ½ zucchini, chopped
- 2 tablespoon extra virgin olive oil
- 4 cloves of garlic, minced
- One handful fresh parsley, finely chopped
- 1/8 teaspoon cayenne powder
- 2 tablespoon tamari or soy sauce

Instructions:
1. Add some water to a frying pan and bring it to boil.
2. Add in the veggies and cook for 2 minutes on high heat.
3. Drain veggies and set aside.
4. Add olive oil, garlic, parsley, and cayenne and cook for 2 minutes.
5. Add in rice and drained vegetables and cook for 1 minute.
6. Serve and enjoy.

Nutrition Facts Per Serving
Calories 179, Total Fat 7.9g, Saturated Fat 1.2g, Total Carbs 24.5g, Protein 4.5g, Sugar:2.4g, Fiber:2.7g, Sodium:522mg, Potassium 330mg

Teriyaki Stir Fry

Prep time: 10 minutes, cook time: 15 minutes; Serves 5

Ingredients:
- 6 small sweet red peppers, chopped
- 1 onion, chopped
- 1 small head broccoli, chopped
- 1 cup carrots, shredded
- 1 cup jasmine rice, cooked
- 1(12 ounces) package frozen shelled edamame
- 2 cloves garlic, minced
- 2 teaspoon ground ginger
- Salt & pepper, to taste
- 4 stalks green onion, chopped for garnish
- Sprinkle of sesame seeds, for garnish
- Few splashes of vegetable broth, for finishing
- Few dollops homemade teriyaki sauce, for garnish

Instructions:
1. Add red peppers, onions, broccoli, and carrots to a saucepan and sauté for 5 minutes over medium heat.
2. Stir in all the remaining ingredients and sauté for about 3 minutes.
3. Serve with jasmine rice and enjoy it.

Nutrition Facts Per Serving
Calories 291, Total Fat 4.1g, Saturated Fat 0.4g, Total Carbs 53.5g, Protein 12.4g, Sugar:11.3g, Fiber:7.6g, Sodium:35mg, Potassium807mg

Spinach and Mushroom Pasta

Prep time: 10 minutes, cook time: 15 minutes; Serves 4

Ingredients:

- 8 ounces whole-wheat spaghetti
- 1 teaspoon olive oil, plus 1 tablespoon
- 2 cups sliced mushrooms
- Salt and freshly ground black pepper
- 4 garlic cloves, minced
- 4 cups baby spinach
- 2 teaspoons freshly squeezed lemon juice
- ¼ teaspoon red pepper flakes
- ¼ teaspoon dried oregano
- 2 tablespoons fresh basil leaves cut into thin strips
- 2 tablespoons pine nuts
- ¼ cup shredded Parmesan cheese

Instructions:

1. Bring a large pot of water to a boil.
2. Cook the spaghetti according to the package directions, then drain.
3. In a large skillet, heat one teaspoon of olive oil over medium heat. Add the mushrooms and season with salt and pepper.
4. Cook over medium heat for ten minutes, stirring occasionally. Add the garlic and spinach and cook for 3 minutes more. Add the lemon juice.
5. Add the spaghetti and season with more salt and pepper. Add the red pepper flakes, oregano, and basil and stir until combined.
6. Top with the remaining one tablespoon of olive oil, the pine nuts, and the Parmesan cheese just before serving.

Nutrition Facts Per Serving

Calories 277, Total Fat 10g, Total Carbs 37g, Protein 12g, Sugar:3g, Fiber:6g, Sodium:425mg

Creamy Spinach Pasta

Prep time: 10 minutes, cook time: 15 minutes; Serves 6

Ingredients:

- 8 oz dry pasta, cooked
- 2 tablespoon olive oil
- 1½ tablespoon garlic, minced
- 3 tablespoon flour
- 1 teaspoon onion powder
- ½ teaspoon salt
- 1½ teaspoon dried oregano
- 1 cup cashew cream
- 1 cup unsweetened milk
- 1 can diced tomatoes

Instructions:

1. Add garlic to a skillet and sauté for 1 minute.
2. Sauté for 1 minute.
3. Add in flour, onion powder, and salt and sauté for a minute.
4. Add in cream, milk, oregano, and parmesan and bring to a boil, stirring constantly.
5. Whisk for a minute then add tomato in it. Stir in pasta and combine well.
6. Serve and enjoy.

Nutrition Facts Per Serving

Calories 209, Total Fat 4g, Saturated Fat 1g, Total Carbs 30g, Protein 6g, Sugar:2g, Fiber:0g, Sodium:2mg, Potassium239mg

Red Pepper Pasta

Prep time: 10 minutes, cook time: 50 minutes; Serves 4

Ingredients:

- 4 red bell peppers
- 1 lb Roma tomatoes
- 10 garlic cloves, peeled
- 1 lb whole-wheat pasta
- 1 tablespoon olive oil
- Salt to taste

Instructions:

1. Preheat the oven to 400°F. Line a baking sheet with parchment paper.
2. Cut the bell peppers in half lengthwise and remove the seeds. Place the bell peppers cut-side down on the prepared baking sheet.
3. Cut the tomatoes in half. Place them and the garlic in a large baking dish.
4. Roast the bell peppers, tomatoes, and garlic for 10 to 15 minutes until the peppers have started to blacken.
5. Set the tomatoes aside to cool. Using tongs, carefully transfer the bell peppers to a large bowl, cover with aluminum foil, and let sit for 15 minutes.
6. In the meantime, bring a large pot of water to a boil. Add the pasta and cook according to the package directions, then drain.
7. When they are cool enough to handle, peel the skin off the peppers and tomatoes. The skin should slide off or use your hands to pull it off.
8. Place the peeled peppers, peeled tomatoes, garlic, and olive oil in a blender or food processor. Blend until smooth then season with salt.
9. Top the pasta with the red pepper sauce and serve immediately.

Nutrition Facts Per Serving

Calories 276, Total Fat 5g, Total Carbs 53g, Protein 10g, Sugar:9g, Fiber:9g, Sodium:86mg

CHAPTER
9

Dessert Recipes

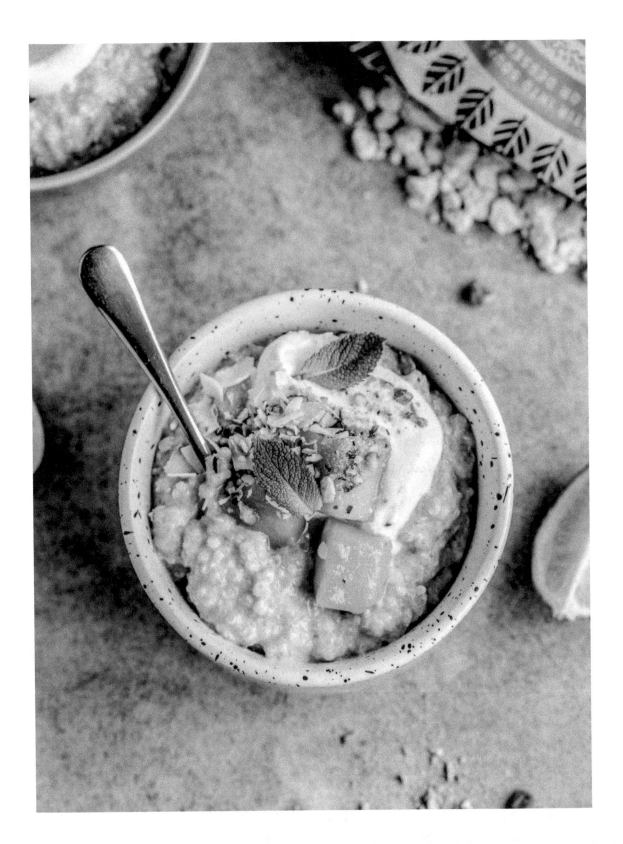

Chocolate Hummus

Prep time: 10 minutes, Chill time: 1 Hour; Serves 7

Ingredients:

- 1 (15-ounce) can of unsalted chickpeas, rinsed and drained
- 1 tablespoon coconut oil
- ⅓ Cup Nutella
- ¼ cup of chocolate coconut milk
- 2 tablespoons cocoa powder
- ¼ teaspoon of sea salt

Instructions:

1. Put the chickpeas, coconut oil, Nutella, chocolate coconut milk, cocoa powder, and salt in a blender.
2. Blend until smooth, then refrigerate for an hour, until chilled.
3. Serve cold with your favorite fruits, like strawberries or peaches.

Nutrition Facts Per Serving

Calories 268, Total Fat 14g, Saturated Fat 6g, Total Carbs 30g, Protein 6g, Sugar:19g, Fiber:5g, Sodium:101mg

Coconut-Quinoa Pudding

Prep time: 5 minutes, cook time: 20 minutes; Serves 6

Ingredients:

- 2 cups almond milk
- 1½ cups quinoa
- 1 cup light coconut milk
- ½ cup maple syrup
- Pinch salt
- 1 teaspoon pure vanilla extract

Instructions:

1. In a large saucepan, heat the almond milk, quinoa, coconut milk, maple syrup, salt, and vanilla over medium-high heat.
2. Bring the quinoa mixture to a boil and then reduce the heat to low.
3. Simmer until the quinoa is tender, frequently stirring, about 20 minutes.
4. Remove the pudding from the heat.
5. Serve warm.

Nutrition Facts Per Serving

Calories 249, Total Fat 6g, Saturated Fat 2g, Total Carbs 42g, Protein 6g, Fiber:3g, Sodium:161mg

No-Bake Cookie Dough

Prep time: 10 minutes, Chill time: 1 hour; serves 7

Ingredients:
- 1 (15-ounce) can no-salt-added chickpeas, rinsed and drained
- ¼ cup of your favorite nut butter
- 3 tablespoons brown sugar
- 1 tablespoon vanilla extract
- ⅓ Cup chocolate chips

Instructions:
1. Place the chickpeas, nut butter, brown sugar, and vanilla in a blender or food processor then blend until smooth.
2. Transfer to a mixing bowl. Fold in the chocolate chips. Cover and refrigerate for an hour.
3. Serve cold and enjoy by the spoonful or as a spread between two graham crackers.

Nutrition Facts Per Serving

Calories 195, Total Fat 10g, Saturated Fat 4g, Total Carbs 22g, Protein 7g, Sugar:9g, Fiber:3g, Sodium:54mg

Baked Pears

Prep time: 5 minutes, cook time: 20 minutes; Serves 4

Ingredients:
- 4 ripe pears, halved
- 1 tablespoon olive oil
- 1 tablespoon pure maple syrup
- 2 teaspoons ground cinnamon
- 1 cup Greek yogurt
- ½ cup of your favorite granola
- Sea salt

Instructions:
1. Preheat the oven to 375°F then line a baking sheet with aluminum foil or parchment paper.
2. Using a spoon, scoop out the center of each pear half, making sure to remove the seeds. Transfer the pears cut-side up to the baking sheet.
3. Brush the pears with the olive oil. Add a drizzle of maple syrup and a dash of cinnamon to each half — Bake for 20 minutes.
4. Once done baking, carefully transfer two pear halves to each plate.
5. Add a few tablespoons of yogurt to the centers, followed by a hearty spoonful of granola. Sprinkle with a dash of sea salt before serving.

Nutrition Facts Per Serving

Calories234, Total Fat 5g, Saturated Fat 2g, Total Carbs, Protein 7g, Sugar:27g, Fiber:6g, Sodium:90mg

Easy Mango Sorbet

Prep time: 10 minutes, Freeze time: 5 hours; Serves 4

Ingredients:

- ½ cup of coconut milk
- ½ cup of sugar
- 1 (12-ounce) bag frozen mango chunks
- 1 tablespoon freshly squeezed lime juice
- Fresh mint, for garnish (optional)

Instructions:

1. In a small saucepan over low heat, make syrup by heating the coconut milk.
2. Add the sugar and let it dissolve completely, often stirring, about 2 minutes.
3. Add the syrup to a blender along with the frozen mango and lime juice.
4. Blend until smooth, and then transfer to a loaf pan or baking dish.
5. Cover and place in the freezer for 5 hours, or until ready to serve.
6. With an ice cream scoop or tablespoon, scoop out the sorbet into four small bowls.
7. Top with the mint or basil before serving, if desired.

Nutrition Facts Per Serving

Calories 211, Total Fat 6g, Saturated Fat5g, Total Carbs 39g, Protein 1g, Sugar:37g, Fiber:2g, Sodium:0mg

Grilled Peaches

Prep time: 10 minutes, cook time: 10 minutes; Serves 4

Ingredients:

- ½ cup heavy (whipping) cream
- 1 tablespoon brown sugar
- ½ teaspoon vanilla extract
- ¼ teaspoon ground cardamom
- 4 ripe peaches, halved and pitted
- 1 tablespoon grapeseed oil
- 1½ tablespoons honey, for drizzling

Instructions:

1. Whip the heavy cream using a mixer then add the sugar, vanilla, and cardamom and beat on high speed until peaks form. Chill in the refrigerator until needed.
2. Heat your grill or stove-top grill pan to medium heat. Brush the peach halves with oil to prevent sticking, then place flat-side down to sear.
3. Grill for five minutes, or until grill marks form, then remove and place two halves in each serving bowl. Drizzle with the honey.
4. Remove the whipped cream from the fridge and divide it evenly among the bowls. Serve immediately.

Nutrition Facts Per Serving

Calories 231, Total Fat 15g, Saturated Fat 7g, Total Carbs 25g, Protein 2g, Sugar:23g, Fiber:2g, Sodium:15mg

Peach Popsicles

Prep time: 10 minutes, Freeze time: 5 hours; Serves 7

Ingredients:
- 1 (14-ounce) can light coconut milk
- 2 peaches, peeled, pitted, and roughly chopped
- ¼ cup honey
- Pinch cinnamon

Instructions:
1. In a blender, blend the coconut milk, peaches, honey, and cinnamon until smooth.
2. Pour the mixture into ice pop molds and freeze for about 5 hours.
3. Enjoy.

Nutrition Facts Per Serving
Calories 80, Total Fat 3g, Saturated Fat 3g, Total Carbs 13g, Protein 0g, Fiber:1g, Sodium: 4mg

Lemon Curd

Prep time: 10 minutes, Chill time: 2 hours, cook time: 5 minutes; Serves 8

Ingredients:
- 1 large egg
- 3 large egg yolks
- ½ cup of sugar
- ⅓ cup of freshly squeezed lemon juice
- 2 tablespoons unsalted butter
- Pinch salt
- 1½ tablespoons heavy (whipping) cream

Instructions:
1. In a small saucepan, whisk the egg, egg yolks, and sugar together. Once combined, turn the burner to low heat and whisk in the lemon juice, butter, and salt.
2. Slowly heat until the butter melts, and the mixture starts to thicken.
3. Heat to 170°F (about 5 minutes), and verify using a kitchen thermometer.
4. Remove from the heat, stir in the cream, and transfer to a mason jar.
5. Cover and chill for at least 2 hours before serving to allow the curd to set.

Nutrition Facts Per Serving
Calories 161, Total Fat 6g, Saturated Fat 3.5g, Total Carbs 26g, Protein 2g, Sugar:25g, Fiber:0g, Sodium:55 mg

Melon-Lime Sorbet

Prep time: 10 minutes, Freeze time: 6 Hours; Serves 8

Ingredients:

- 1 small honeydew melon, peeled, seeded, and cut into 1-inch chunks
- 1 small cantaloupe, peeled, seeded, and cut into 1-inch pieces
- 2 tablespoons honey
- 2 tablespoons freshly squeezed lime juice
- Pinch cinnamon
- Water as needed

Instructions:

1. Spread the honeydew and cantaloupe out on a baking sheet lined with parchment paper and put it in the freezer for 6 hours until frozen.
2. In a food processor, add the frozen melon chunks and the honey, lime juice, and cinnamon.
3. Pulse until smooth, adding water if needed to purée the melon.
4. Transfer the mixture to a container and place in the freezer until set, about 30 minutes.

Nutrition Facts Per Serving

Calories 96, Total Fat 0g, Saturated Fat 0g, Total Carbs 25g, Protein 2g, Fiber:2g, Sodium:39mg

Raspberry S'mores

Prep time: 5 minutes, cook time: 5 minutes; Serves 4

Ingredients:

- 4 graham crackers
- 2 tablespoons Homemade Lemon Curd
- 2 tablespoons raspberry jam
- 4 white chocolate squares
- 4 jumbo marshmallows

Instructions:

1. To make each s'more, break a graham cracker in half to form two squares.
2. Spread the lemon curd onto one half and the raspberry jam on the other half.
3. Place the white chocolate square on one half.
4. Toast the marshmallows over a grill.
5. Once heated, place on top of the white chocolate square and top the s'more with the other half of the graham cracker.
6. Serve immediately.

Nutrition Facts Per Serving

Calories 311, Total Fat 8.5g, Saturated Fat4.5g, Total Carbs 56g, Protein 3g, Sugar:38g, Fiber:0g, Sodium:215mg

CHAPTER
10

Beans and Legumes Recipes

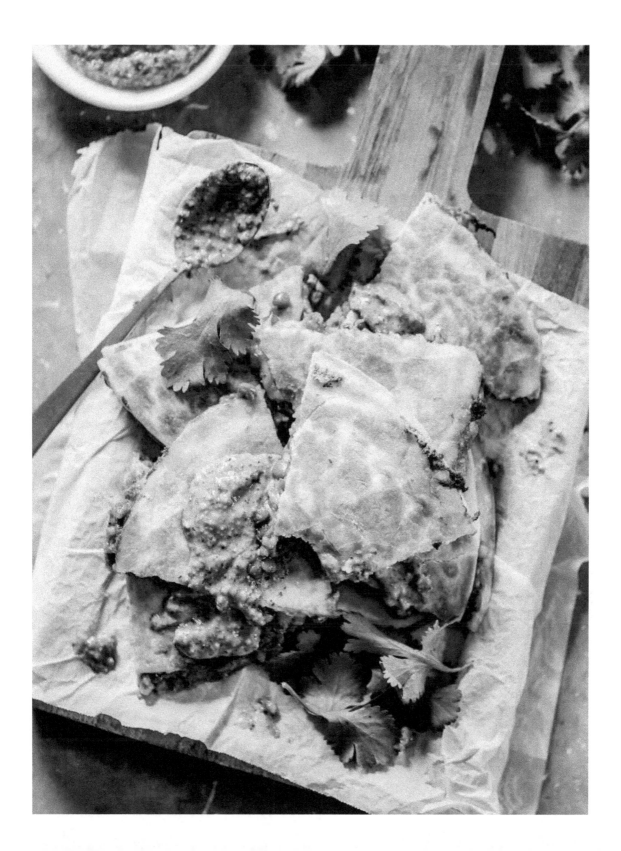

Lentil Quesadillas

Prep time: 10 minutes, cook time: 15 minutes; Serves 4

Ingredients:
- 4 (6-inch) whole-wheat tortillas
- 1 tablespoon olive oil
- 1 (15-ounce) can lentils, drained and rinsed
- 1 yellow bell pepper, seeded and finely chopped
- 1 tomato, diced
- ½ cup feta cheese, crumbled

Instructions:
1. Preheat the oven to 450°F. Line a baking sheet with parchment paper.
2. Place two tortillas on the baking sheet and brush with olive oil
3. Flip the tortillas over, so the oiled side is on the bottom.
4. Evenly divide the lentils between the tortillas and spread them out.
5. Evenly divide the bell pepper, tomato, and feta between the tortillas.
6. Top with the remaining tortillas and brush the tops with oil.
7. Bake the tortillas in the oven, flipping once, until they are crispy and lightly browned, about 15 minutes total.
8. Cut the quesadillas into quarters and serve.

Nutrition Facts Per Serving
Calories 397, Total Fat13g, Saturated Fat 4g, Total Carbs 54g, Protein 17g, Fiber:12g, Sodium:482mg

Navy Bean Broccoli Toss

Prep time: 10 minutes, cook time: 15 minutes; Serves 4

Ingredients:
- 2 tablespoons olive oil
- ½ sweet onion, finely chopped
- 2 teaspoons minced garlic
- 2 anchovy fillets packed in oil
- 2 (15-ounce) cans navy beans, drained and rinsed
- 1 broccoli head cut into small florets
- 1 red bell pepper, seeded and diced
- Juice and zest of 1 lemon
- Sea salt and black pepper for seasoning

Instructions:
1. In a large saucepan, heat the olive oil over medium-high heat.
2. Sauté the onion and garlic until softened, about 3 minutes.
3. Add the anchovies and sauté 1 minute more.
4. Stir in the beans and sauté until heated through about 6 minutes.
5. Stir in the broccoli, bell pepper, lemon juice, and lemon zest and sauté until the broccoli is tender-crisp about 5 minutes
6. Season with salt and pepper and serve.

Nutrition Facts Per Serving
Calories 416, Total Fat 10g, Saturated Fat 1g, Total Carbs 60g, Protein 25g, Fiber:15g, Sodium: 1467mg

White Bean Stew and Cauliflower

Prep time: 10 minutes, cook time: 30 minutes; Serves 4

Ingredients:

- 1 tablespoon olive oil
- 1 cup thinly sliced yellow onion
- 1 tablespoon garlic paste or minced garlic
- ½ jalapeño pepper, minced
- 1 teaspoon kosher salt
- Pinch freshly ground black pepper
- 2 cups chopped cauliflower
- 4 cups vegetable broth
- 2 cups canned cannellini beans

Instructions:

1. Heat the olive oil in a large pot over medium-high heat.
2. Add the onion, garlic paste, jalapeño, salt, and black pepper, and cook until the vegetables soften and are very fragrant about 10 minutes.
3. Mix in the cauliflower, and then add the vegetable broth and beans.
4. Bring to a simmer and cook until the cauliflower is tender forabout20 minutes.

Nutrition Facts Per Serving

Calories 131, Total Fat 4g, Total Carbs 20g, Protein 6g, Sugar:6g, Fiber:6g, Sodium:758mg

Lentil Potato Salad

Prep time: 10 minutes, cook time: 25 minutes; Serves 2

Ingredients:

- ½ cup lentils
- 8 fingerling potatoes
- 1 cup thinly sliced scallions
- ¼ cup of halved cherry tomatoes
- ¼ cup Lemon Vinaigrette
- Kosher salt, and freshly ground black pepper to taste

Instructions:

1. Bring 2 cups of water to a simmer in a small pot and add the lentils. Cover and simmer until the lentils are tender (about 20 minutes). Drain and set aside to cool.
2. While the lentils are cooking, bring a medium pot of well-salted water to a boil and add the potatoes. Reduce the heat to a simmer and cook for about 15 minutes, or until the potatoes are tender. Drain. Once cool enough to handle, slice, or halve the potatoes.
3. Place the lentils on a serving plate and top with the potatoes, scallions, and tomatoes.
4. Drizzle with the vinaigrette and season with the salt and pepper.

Nutrition Facts Per Serving

Calories 400, Total Fat 26g, Total Carbs 39g, Protein 7g, Sugar:5g, Fiber:6g, Sodium:1200mg

Tahini Falafels

Prep time: 10 minutes, cook time: 30 minutes; Serves 4

Ingredients:
- 2 cups broccoli florets
- 2 cups dry chickpeas, cooked
- ½ cup dry black beans, cooked
- 1 garlic clove (minced)
- 2 teaspoons cumin
- 1 teaspoon olive oil
- ½ teaspoon lemon juice
- ½ teaspoon paprika
- ¼ teaspoon turmeric
- Dash of salt
- 2 tablespoon tahini

Instructions:
1. Preheat the oven to 400° F.
2. Meanwhile, place the broccoli florets in a large skillet and drizzle them with olive oil and salt.
3. Roast the broccoli over medium-high heat until the florets are tender and brown for 5 to 10 minutes; set aside and allow cooling a little.
4. Place the cooled broccoli with all the remaining ingredients—except the tahini—into a food processor. Blend on low for 2-3 minutes, until most large lumps are gone.
5. Line a baking pan with parchment paper. Press the falafel dough into eight equal-sized patties, and place them evenly-spaced apart on the parchment.
6. Bake the falafels until they are brown and crisp on the outside, for roughly 10 to 15 minutes. Make sure to flip them halfway through to ensure even cooking.
7. Serve with tahini as a topping, or let the falafel cool down and store for later.

Nutrition Facts Per Serving
Calories 220, Total Fat7.3g, Total Carbs 28g, Protein 10.5g, Sugar: 3.9g, Fiber: 8g,)

Black Bean & Quinoa Burgers

Prep time: 10 minutes, cook time: 35 minutes; Serves 3

Ingredients:
- 2 tbsp. olive oil
- ½ chopped red onion
- ¼ cup bell pepper, seeded and chopped
- 2 tablespoons garlic, minced
- 1 tsp. salt
- 1 tsp. pepper
- 1 cup dry black beans, cooked
- ½ cup dry quinoa
- ½ cup whole wheat flour
- ½ tsp. Red pepper flakes
- ½ tsp. paprika
- 5 large leaves of lettuce
- Roasted sesame seeds (optional)

Instructions:
1. Heat 1 tablespoon of the olive oil in a frying pan over medium-high heat and then add the onions, bell peppers, garlic, salt, and pepper.
2. Sauté until the ingredients begin to soften, for about 5 minutes.
3. Remove the pan from the heat and let it cool down for about 10 minutes.
4. Once the veggies have cooled down, put them in a food processor along with the cooked beans, quinoa, flour, and remaining spices; pulse until it's a chunky mixture.

5. Lay a pan covered with parchment paper and form the blended mixture into six evenly-sized patties.
6. Place the patties on the pan and place them in the freezer for about 5 minutes to prevent crumbling.
7. Heat the remaining oil in a frying pan over high heat and add the burgers. Cook the patties until they have browned, for about 2-3 minutes per side.
8. Serve each burger wrapped in a lettuce leaf (or burger bun) and, if desired, top with the optional roasted sesame seeds.

Calories 200, Total Fat 10.6g, Saturated Fat, Total Carbs 40.5g, Net Carbs, Protein 9.5g, Sugar:2.8g, Fiber:8.2g,)

Red Beans & Rice

Prep time: 10 minutes, cook time: 25 minutes; Serves 4

Ingredients:

- 1½ cups of dry red beans
- 2 tablespoon olive oil
- ½ cup sweet onion, chopped
- ½ cup celery ribs, diced
- ½ cup green bell pepper, chopped
- 1 large head of cauliflower (or 3 cups frozen cauliflower rice)
- 1 tablespoon garlic, minced
- 2 cups of water
- 2 teaspoon cumin
- 1 teaspoon paprika
- 1 teaspoon chili powder
- ½ teaspoon basil
- ½ teaspoon parsley flakes
- ½ teaspoon black pepper
- ¼ cup parsley
- ¼ cup basil

Instructions:
1. Heat the olive oil in a large frying pan over medium-high heat.
2. Add the onion, celery, and green pepper and sauté until everything has softened in about 7 minutes.
3. Place the cauliflower into a food processor. Pulse until it resembles rice in about 15 seconds.
4. Add the cups of water, rice, beans, and remaining ingredients to the pan.
5. Mix all the ingredients until wholly distributed and cook until the cauliflower rice is soft, about 10 minutes.
6. Serve into bowls and, if desired, garnish with the optional parsley or basil, or store to enjoy later!

Calories 235, Total Fat 8.3g, Saturated Fat, Total Carbs 32.3g, Protein 7.9g, Sugar: 2.2g, Fiber:7.3g,)

Lentil with Paprika

Prep time: 10 minutes, cook time: 45 minutes; Serves 5

Ingredients:

- Splash water
- 1½ cups onion, diced
- 1 cup carrot, cut
- 5 cloves garlic, minced
- 1½ teaspoon dried thyme
- 1½ teaspoon smoked paprika
- 1 teaspoon Dijon mustard
- ¾ teaspoon of sea salt
- Freshly ground black pepper, to taste
- 2 cups French lentils, rinsed
- 2 cups vegetable stock
- 5 cups of water
- ¼ cup tomato paste
- 1 bay leaf

Instructions:

1. Heat a large pot over medium heat.
2. Add all ingredients in it to the pot and cook for ten minutes, stirring occasionally.
3. Increase heat and bring it to a boil.
4. Once it boils, let it simmer for about 40 minutes.
5. Remove bay leaf.
6. Serve and enjoy.

Nutrition Facts Per Serving

Calories 109, Total Fat0.9g, Saturated Fat0.5g, Total Carbs 26.1g, Protein 5.7g, Sugar: 8.6g, Fiber: 8.3g, Sodium: 200mg, Potassium 431mg

Tempeh with Fried Rice

Prep time: 10 minutes, cook time: 2 hours 20 minutes; Serves 4

Ingredients:

- 2 (8-ounce) packages tempeh
- ½ cup low-sodium soy sauce, divided
- 2 tablespoons maple syrup
- 2 tablespoons avocado oil, divided
- 3 cups cooked brown rice, cold or room temperature
- 1 egg
- 1 cup broccoli florets
- ½ cup corn kernels
- ½ cup peas
- 1 garlic clove, minced
- 1 teaspoon grated fresh ginger

Instructions:

1. Cut the tempeh into ¼-inch strips. Place them in a shallow dish large enough to hold them in a single layer.
2. In a small bowl, whisk together ¼ cup of soy sauce and the maple syrup.
3. Drizzle the sauce over the tempeh, turning each piece to ensure it coats evenly.
4. Cover with plastic wrap and marinate for at least 2 hours, or overnight, in the refrigerator.
5. In a large nonstick skillet, heat one tablespoon of avocado oil over medium heat. Place the marinated tempeh in a single layer in the skillet. (You may need to cook it in batches.)
6. Cook for 5 to 7 minutes, letting it brown before flipping over. Continue to cook on the other side for 3 to 5 minutes until browned and crispy.
7. Remove the tempeh and set aside.

8. Add the remaining one tablespoon of avocado oil to the skillet, then add the rice and stir well.
9. Push the rice to one side and add the egg to the other side of the skillet. Raise the heat to be high and scramble the egg into the rice.
10. Add the broccoli, corn, and peas and cook for 2 to 3 minutes if fresh (5 to 6 minutes if frozen) until the veggies are brightly colored and begin to soften. Add the remaining ¼ cup of soy sauce and the garlic and ginger and cook for another minute.
11. Return the tempeh to the pan and toss it with the rice and vegetables until the tempeh heats through.

Nutrition Facts Per Serving
Calories 619, Total Fat 18g, Total Carbs 89g, Protein 32g, Sugar:10g, Fiber:6g, Sodium:989mg

Stuffed Bell Peppers

Prep time: 10 minutes, cook time: 30 minutes; Serves 6

Ingredients:
- 3 bell peppers (red or yellow, seeded)
- 2 tbsp. olive oil
- 1 sweet onion, chopped
- 2 tbsp. garlic, minced
- 1 tablespoon Parsley
- ½ tablespoon dried basil
- ½ cup kale, chopped,
- 2 tbsp. water
- 1 cup dry black beans, cooked
- ½ cup dry chickpeas, cooked
- ½ cup dry quinoa, cooked
- Salt and pepper to taste

Instructions:
1. Preheat the oven to 400°F
2. Slice the bell peppers in half and remove (and discard) the seeds, stem, and placenta.
3. Place the peppers skin down on a large baking sheet and drizzle with one tablespoon of the olive oil, making sure the bell peppers are fully covered — Bake the bell pepper halves for 10 minutes, or until the skins begin to soften.
4. While the peppers are baking, heat 1 tablespoon of olive oil in a frying pan over medium heat. Add the onion, cook until translucent (around 5 minutes), and stir in the garlic, parsley, basil, kale, and water.
5. Sauté for about 2 minutes and mix in the cooked quinoa, chickpeas, and black beans until warmed through.
6. Season the mixture to taste, stir for few minutes, and remove from heat.
7. Spoon the filling equally into the pepper halves and place them back into the oven for about 10 minutes.
8. Remove the filled bell peppers from the oven when the peppers are soft and fragrant.
9. Store for later, or serve right away and enjoy!

Nutrition Facts Per Serving
Calories 171, Total Fat 5.2g, Saturated Fat, Total Carbs 24.7g, Net Carbs, Protein 6.3g, Sugar:4.8g, Fiber:5.9g)

Conclusion

Thank you again for downloading this book! I hope the book gave you insight on the pescatarian diet, as well as offer you tips and recipes that you will enjoy very much.

This diet has helped such a significant number of people throughout the years. I guarantee that if you stay consistent, this diet will work for you. I do not doubt that these recipes can assist you in reaching your health or fitness goals. By adopting this diet, you will feel more energized and productive throughout your day, sleep better at night, and live a more healthy life. Make little progress each day towards a full pescatarian diet, and before you know it, you will be all in!

Hopefully, you have delighted in the recipes that I have compiled for you here. I tried to ensure that there is something for every taste, budget, and occasion. The recipes are quite easy to prepare, and the ingredients all accessible at your local grocery store.
I am confident that trying out these recipes will make you appreciate the simplicity, assortment, and versatility of seafood and a pescatarian diet in general.

Bon Appétit!

Appendix 1: Measurement Conversion Chart

VOLUME EQUIVALENTS(DRY)

US STANDARD	METRIC (APPROXIMATE)
1/8 teaspoon	0.5 mL
1/4 teaspoon	1 mL
1/2 teaspoon	2 mL
3/4 teaspoon	4 mL
1 teaspoon	5 mL
1 tablespoon	15 mL
1/4 cup	59 mL
1/2 cup	118 mL
3/4 cup	177 mL
1 cup	235 mL
2 cups	475 mL
3 cups	700 mL
4 cups	1 L

WEIGHT EQUIVALENTS

US STANDARD	METRIC (APPROXIMATE)
1 ounce	28 g
2 ounces	57 g
5 ounces	142 g
10 ounces	284 g
15 ounces	425 g
16 ounces (1 pound)	455 g
1.5 pounds	680 g
2 pounds	907 g

VOLUME EQUIVALENTS(LIQUID)

US STANDARD	US STANDARD (OUNCES)	METRIC (APPROXIMATE)
2 tablespoons	1 fl.oz.	30 mL
1/4 cup	2 fl.oz.	60 mL
1/2 cup	4 fl.oz.	120 mL
1 cup	8 fl.oz.	240 mL
1 1/2 cup	12 fl.oz.	355 mL
2 cups or 1 pint	16 fl.oz.	475 mL
4 cups or 1 quart	32 fl.oz.	1 L
1 gallon	128 fl.oz.	4 L

TEMPERATURES EQUIVALENTS

FAHRENHEIT(F)	CELSIUS(C) (APPROXIMATE)
225 °F	107 °C
250 °F	120 °C
275 °F	135 °C
300 °F	150 °C
325 °F	160 °C
350 °F	180 °C
375 °F	190 °C
400 °F	205 °C
425 °F	220 °C
450 °F	235 °C
475 °F	245 °C
500 °F	260 °C

Appendix 2: Recipe Index

Printed in the USA
CPSIA information can be obtained
at www.ICGtesting.com